Metabolic and
Nutritional Diseases

LIBRARY OF VETERINARY PRACTICE

EDITORS

C. J. PRICE MA, VetMB, MRCVS
The Veterinary Hospital
49 Cambridge Street
Aylesbury, Bucks

P. G. C. BEDFORD BVetMed, PhD, DVOphthal, FRCVS
Royal Veterinary College
Hawkshead Lane, North Mymms, Hatfield, Herts

J. B. SUTTON JP, MRCVS
2 Friarswood Road
Newcastle-under-Lyme, Staffs

LIBRARY OF VETERINARY PRACTICE

Metabolic and
Nutritional Diseases of Cattle

The Late J. M. PAYNE
'Southlands'
Garden Close Lane
Newbury
Berks RG14 6PP

BLACKWELL SCIENTIFIC PUBLICATIONS

OXFORD LONDON EDINBURGH

BOSTON MELBOURNE

© 1989 by
Blackwell Scientific Publications
Editorial offices:
Osney Mead, Oxford OX2 oEL
   (*Orders*: Tel: 0865 240201)
8 John Street, London WCIN 2ES
23 Ainslie Place, Edinburgh EH3 6AJ
3 Cambridge Center, Suite 208
   Cambridge, Massachusetts 02142,
   USA
107 Barry Street, Carlton
   Victoria 3053, Australia

First published 1989

Set by Macmillan India Ltd
Printed and bound in Great Britain
by The Alden Press, Oxford

DISTRIBUTORS

USA
   Year Book Medical Publishers
   200 North LaSalle Street
   Chicago, Illinois 60601
   (*Orders*: Tel: (312) 726-9733)

Canada
   The C. V. Mosby Company
   5240 Finch Avenue East
   Scarborough, Ontario
   (*Orders*: Tel: 416 298-1588)

Australia
   Blackwell Scientific Publications
   (Australia) Pty Ltd
   107 Barry Street
   Carlton, Victoria 3053
   (*Orders*: Tel: (03) 347-0300)

British Library
Cataloguing in Publication Data

Payne, J M
   Metabolic and nutritional diseases of
cattle.
   1. Livestock. Cattle. Metabolic
disorders.
   Nutritional disorders
   I. Title.   II. Series.
   636.2'089639

   ISBN 0-632-01969-7

Contents

Foreword

Like other books in the Library of Veterinary Practice Series, *Metabolic and Nutritional Diseases of Cattle* is designed to supply up-to-date information relevant to the subject in a concise format so that specific facts can be located quickly and easily.

Professor Payne, an acknowledged expert on this subject, has produced a book which fulfils this objective admirably. Tragically, he died suddenly when the manuscript was almost complete. The editor and publishers are greatly indebted to his widow, Sylvia Payne, herself a PhD, who so kindly and efficiently stepped into the breach by completing the final chapters and reading the proofs.

I hope that students and practitioners alike will find the information collected here of invaluable help in this important aspect of bovine medicine.

J. B. Sutton

1 / Introduction

General concepts

The term *metabolic disease* conveys various meanings depending on how the reader interprets the concepts involved. At its simplest the term refers merely to the three clinical syndromes: parturient hypocalcaemia (milk fever), hypomagnesaemia (grass tetany), and ketosis (slow fever or acetonaemia). All three share common features. The underlying cause of each is an upset of metabolism resulting in a failure of homeostasis. In the case of milk fever, calcium metabolism is upset, for grass tetany magnesium metabolism is upset and for ketosis glucose and energy metabolism is upset. The homeostasis of calcium, magnesium and glucose needs close control because when concentrations in the blood deviate far from the normal, then dramatic changes in physiology ensue. In the case of calcium, magnesium and glucose the most obvious defects occur in the function of the brain and the central nervous system.

The internal environment of the body fluids remains constant, not because of a static level of its constituents but because of a balanced and continuous inflow and outflow of metabolites. If a change in the rate of either the inflow or the outflow fails to be met by an equal and opposite counter-effect then the dynamic equilibrium of the system changes with the inevitable result of a change in concentration and eventually a breakdown of homeostasis.

Several factors conspire to preserve the equilibrium. First, animals have evolved complicated endocrinological systems of control. This is certainly so for calcium and glucose. Calcium is controlled by a complicated mechanism involving two hormones, parathormone and calcitonin. Similarly, glucose is controlled by insulin and glucagon. In contrast, magnesium seems to have no direct hormonal control and consequently hypomagnesaemia supervenes fairly easily. Second, the stability of the inflow/outflow system of equilibrium depends largely on the actual quantity of metabolite circulating in the body fluids, the so-called 'pool size'. Thus a rapid throughput with a small 'pool size' presents an inherently unstable and dangerous situation, liable to violent fluctuation. Table 1.1 illustrates this point. A high-yielding cow has calcium throughput rates of 34 g of calcium per day with only 3 g of immediately usable reserves. Similarly, magnesium has a turnover of 4 g per day with a pool size of only 0.75 g. Thus a small change in the rates of inflow or outflow can trigger a swiftly developing catastrophe which is why milk fever and grass tetany are rapidly fatal metabolic disorders. In contrast, sodium and potassium have very large 'pool sizes' relative to their turnover rates and thus any upset in their metabolism develops slowly. In other words there is sufficient buffer in the system to tide the animal over relatively short periods of deficiency without harm.

In general a metabolic disease is defined as *a disturbance of internal homeostasis brought about by an abnormal change in the rate of one or more critical metabolic processes*. It is obvious from this that the metabolites, calcium, magnesium and glucose, represent only three of many metabolites that could be involved in metabolic disease. The subject extends far beyond just milk fever, grass tetany and ketosis. Any metabolic system of the body, including that of water, minerals and trace elements, electrolytes, proteins and energy metabolites, suffers input/output imbalance from time to time with consequent metabolic disorder as revealed by a wide variety of clinical signs.

Even infectious disease caused by pathogens such as bacteria or viruses induces clinical signs by a disturbance of internal homeostasis. Thus, logically, infectious diseases have a claim to be called

Table 1.1 Input–throughput–output relationships for calcium, magnesium, sodium and potassium

Mineral	Input		Throughput		Output	
	Dietary intake (g/day)	Absorbed intake (g/day)	Total reserves (g)	Available reserves (g)	Endogenous loss (g/day)	Milk loss (g/day)
Calcium	100.0	34.0	6000	3.0	8.0	26.0
Magnesium	20.0	4.0	175	0.75	1.5	2.5
Sodium	19.5	19.5	700	35.0	6.5	13.0
Potassium	50.5	50.5	820	185.0	22.5	28.0

metabolic diseases. However, they are excluded because they are not *primarily* induced metabolically. In contrast, deficiency diseases are truly metabolic in the sense that they involve a failure of input of a nutrient or a metabolite to match its output.

Veterinarians use the term metabolic disease quite differently from those working in human medicine. In man, metabolic disease implies some inherent defect in the metabolic constitution of an individual person. This defect could be the congenital absence of a key enzyme which blocks an important metabolic pathway—examples being the so-called 'storage diseases' in which metabolites slowly accumulate because there is no enzyme to relieve their retention. Alternatively there may be an endocrinological failure—lack of insulin in diabetes being a good example. Metabolic diseases like these do occur in cattle (see Chapter 10), but rarely so. Most of the metabolic disorders of cattle result from a breakdown in the animals' capacity to meet the demands of high production coupled with some of the relatively unsuitable feeds commonly offered in modern husbandry. Thus metabolic disease of this kind is, in a sense, man-made and due to the unusual demands we impose on livestock.

This is why the term 'production disease' finds increasing use. It draws attention to the basic cause of the disorder, that in the interests of high production we expose animals to metabolic hazards that they would not normally encounter in the wild.

Principal factors affecting the input and storage of metabolites

The alimentary tract

The alimentary tract of cattle confers unique physiological advantages which tend to become liabilities in some modern husbandry systems. First, their rumen allows them to eat and use fodder which cannot be digested by conventional mammalian digestive enzymes. They can live on roughages and sources of non-protein nitrogen denied to other species. However, rumen fermentation imposes a liability if large quantities of rapidly fermentable carbohydrates are fed. The affected animals die of acute indigestion, or of lactic acid poisoning (see Chapter 6, p. 75). Similarly, the use of urea as a cheap supplement for protein carries the danger of ammonia poisoning if the urea is too rapidly hydrolysed by the bacteria in the rumen.

Second, continuous function of the alimentary tract is vital to maintain the flow of nutrients for lactation. Even brief periods of inappetance or ruminal stasis become potentially fatal. The reason for this is that dairy cattle, being bred for milk production, continue to lactate even though this means that they deplete their bodies of vital reserves. In some metabolic disorders like milk fever just a brief and temporary interruption in gut function induces a potentially fatal deficit of calcium input. In other, more chronic disorders, failure to absorb sufficient nutrient leads to a gradual loss of body substance which must be built back during the dry period to preserve normal lifespan. For example, dairy cows may lose 15% of their skeleton in one lactation and thus bone disease gradually supervenes if no allowance is made for recoupment of reserves during the dry period.

The liver

The liver occupies a central place in metabolism. All the nutrients absorbed from the alimentary tract pass through the liver and many are either converted into other metabolites or are stored as part of a vital reserve. All the glucose needed for lactation is synthesized in the liver. Similarly all the fat mobilized for the energy needs of lactation must be processed in the liver cells. Thus any interruption in the smooth working of liver function must result in disturbance of metabolism. A typical example of this includes fatty change of the liver, which results from the over-rapid mobilization of fat from fat depots in response to the demands of lactation. The accumulation of fat in the liver cells leads to liver failure and eventually to ketosis (see Chapter 6, p. 73).

The liver also stores vital trace elements such as copper. Unfortunately, on diets with a high copper content the stored copper exceeds the safety limits resulting in copper toxicity and massive necrosis of liver cells (see Chapter 11, p. 129).

The skeleton

The vast amounts of mineral, calcium, phosphorus and magnesium stored in the skeleton not only provide the rigid framework

which enables the animal to stand and move about but also a vital reservoir of mineral to tide the animal over periods of relative shortage. The mobilization of bone calcium becomes a limiting factor in the pathogenesis of milk fever (see Chapter 2, p. 16). In the longer term this reservoir of mineral is not inexhaustable. As mentioned above, 15% of it may be removed for the needs of lactation and if this is not built back then painful bone disease ensues.

Another function of bone is the temporary sequestration of toxic trace elements such as fluorine. Unfortunately, long-continued excess intake of fluorine leads to toxicity with severe and painful bone disease.

Husbandry

The metabolic well-being of cattle depends not only on their metabolic constitution and feeding but also on the background soil and pasture of the farm and on the quality of the husbandry which goes into the animals' care. Some soils are deficient in trace elements such as iodine, copper or sodium. This situation worsens as the trace element levels fall still further with continuous cropping unless replacements are put back onto the land. Failure to do this results in increasingly severe outbreaks of pica in which the animals eat bark and soil in vain attempts to correct deficiencies.

Another factor in the pathogenesis of metabolic disorder concerns the excessive use of fertilizer. Extra potassium interferes with the absorption of magnesium and thus predisposes to hypomagnesaemia. Similarly, methaemoglobinaemia results if the animals graze land recently fertilized with nitrate and extra calcium in liming reduces the absorption of copper and zinc. Some excess inputs stem from the natural composition of the soil. For example 'teart' pastures contain excess molybdenum which interferes with the absorption and utilization of copper.

Some deficiencies occur when least expected. Few farmers entertain the possibility of water deficiency except in arid countries. However, inadequate trough space and supply pipes may not cater for cows which tend to drink in batches at certain times of the day only, especially when grazing.

Some metabolic problems follow from intensification of grassland husbandry. For example, this may restrict grazing to only one species of plant. Grazing solely on ryegrass limits the availability of magnesium with consequent increase in liability to grass tetany.

On indoor rations the animals commonly receive all their ration of concentrates in the milking parlours—thus their rumen, which is adapted to a more or less continuous intake, becomes compelled to take in large amounts of highly fermentable material all at once. The rapid fermentation of this predisposes to indigestion and poor appetite (see Chapter 6, p. 75).

A common fallacy is that metabolic disease only occurs in advanced agricultural systems. However, initial attempts at agricultural improvement provoke unforeseen problems. The first reports of metabolic disease in the UK appeared at the end of the eighteenth century at the very beginning of scientific selection for high yields and improved feeding of livestock. Similarly, in present day developing countries agricultural improvements highlight insidious problems that would otherwise have lain dormant. Phosphorus deficiency is a typical example. Animals cope with marginal deficiency but even modest attempts at improved production provoke dramatic clinical signs of bone disease and pica.

Principal factors affecting the output of metabolites

Productivity has risen steadily over the last few decades. How has this come about? First, with skilled breeding and modern husbandry, high-yielding cows became more efficient, their protein conversion rate rising progressively with output. Where is the 'biological ceiling'? Some say up to 4000 gallons of milk per lactation. Although theoretically attainable, many cows break down under the metabolic strain at much lower yields. Second, although high-yielding cows are efficient over one lactation much depends on their overall production over the full lifespan. Cows live only short lives and tend to be culled at about 6 years of age just when they reach maximum production. Early culling is only attractive with high prices for beef which equate with the costly process of rearing calves through to lactation. Third, there is advantage in rapid rearing to reduce the non-productive part of the lifespan. However, these rapidly reared animals are said to have reduced longevity and lifetime productivity. Fourth, economic advantage might be gained with more calves per gestation, i.e. an increased number of twins. How far would the extra metabolic burden of twins be supportable if yields remain high, or climb even further?

Thus many questions can be posed. Future levels of output cannot be forecast with precision and only scientific research can predict the possible ill effects of still further increases in production. Completely new factors may enter the situation. Assume, for instance, that bovine somatotrophin provides a new stimulant for increasing production. What effect will this have on the incidence of existing and possible new metabolic disorders? This is only one of many possible changes that will affect the pattern of metabolic disorder in the future.

2/Disorders associated with mineral metabolism

The minerals calcium, phosphorus and magnesium all play an important part in metabolic and nutritional disease of cattle. They are associated with various types of disorder. Some of these disorders, such as parturient hypocalcaemia or grass tetany (hypomagnesaemia), are acute and rapidly fatal unless treated urgently. Others, such as osteodystrophy, are chronic and take a long time to show clinical signs. They all possess common features especially in aetiology. All follow from imbalances between supply and demand upsetting the delicate control of homeostasis. In the case of parturient hypocalcaemia the sudden demand for calcium by the newly lactating udder overwhelms the capacity of the animal to call up its mineral reserves either from the skeleton or by absorption from the intestines. Similarly, in the case of grass tetany, curtailment in magnesium absorption from the gut for the needs of lactation or tissue growth leads to the rapid onset of hypomagnesaemia and grass tetany. Bone disorders follow a similar though longer-term pattern. Failure to maintain a balanced input and output of mineral into and out of the bones leads either to gradual demineralization or to excessive accretion of new bone or, in very special circumstances, to failure in the remodelling of bone for growth.

Thus, metabolic disorders associated with breakdown of calcium, phosphorus and magnesium metabolism fit into the general concept of production disease. Put simply, they are due to failure of mineral homeostasis in animals confronted with the need to support high growth rate or lactation when fed on diets that are not always entirely suitable or adequate. A knowledge of normal factors controlling mineral homeostasis helps the understanding of ways in which the disorders occur.

Control of mineral homeostasis

Blood concentrations

Only calcium of the three main mineral metabolites comes under firm endocrinological control. Its concentration in the blood, as compared with phosphorus and magnesium, stays constant within very close limits. This shows up clearly in Table 2.1.

Table 2.1 Normal blood concentrations of calcium, phosphorus and magnesium

	Normal mean concentration in blood plasma (mg/100 ml)	Normal range (±2SD)	Coefficient of variation (SD/mean)
Calcium	9.5	8.7–10.3	0.17
Magnesium	2.5	2.0–3.0	0.40
Inorganic phosphorus	6.0	4.3–7.7	0.57

The table reveals quantitatively that blood plasma calcium is at least twice as firmly controlled as magnesium or inorganic phosphorus. Important implications follow. In particular, plasma calcium varies so little from the normal, except in extreme circumstances, that it has no value as a reliable measure of nutritional status. On the other hand, plasma magnesium and inorganic phosphorus concentrations depend on dietary intake and these serve as reliable indicators of dietary adequacy.

The three mineral elements calcium, phosphorus and magnesium circulate in the blood in both simple ionic or in compound ionic forms. Calcium circulates either as calcium ions or protein bound (especially to blood albumin)—approximately half in each form. Small amounts are also complexed to free fatty acids or to phosphate. The calcium ion possesses physiological activity, being especially important for the proper function of cell membranes, in muscular contractility, nervous irritability and blood coagulation. Logically, the estimation of blood calcium should be restricted to the ionized fraction, this being the truly functional form, but the assay proves tedious. Clinicians accept the total calcium value for routine interpretation and in many ways they are justified because, provided blood albumin remains reasonably constant, total calcium values give a valid indication of the ionized fraction.

Blood phosphorus also circulates in ionic or bound form. The usual value quoted in laboratory reports is the unbound anion, inorganic phosphate. The organic or bound fraction seldom receives notice in clinical work, though it includes several forms such as energy-rich compounds and phosphate esters. Phosphorus performs a vital role as a cell constituent especially for energy metabolism. Also, combined with calcium it forms the major structural component of bone.

Blood magnesium resembles calcium in that a proportion of it binds to plasma proteins. In clinical work assays usually measure total magnesium. It plays a vital role in maintaining the normal irritability and function of muscle and nerve cells.

Endocrinological control

Several hormones interact to control calcium concentration but only three—parathyroid hormone, calcitonin and vitamin D_3—act directly.

Parathyroid hormone comes from the parathyroid glands where it is stored as precursor granules in the so-called 'chief cells'. The gland secretes it in response to a fall in blood calcium concentration. Parathyroid hormone stimulates the cells known as osteoclasts in the bone to resorb bone mineral and the calcium thus released raises the blood calcium concentration. Another function of the hormone is to increase the absorption of calcium from the gut, but it does this indirectly by regulating the metabolism of vitamin D_3, which stimulates the synthesis of a calcium-binding protein in the intestinal mucosa, and this in its turn affects calcium absorption. Yet another function of parathyroid hormone works via the kidneys. It allows the secretion of phosphorus in the urine which in turn encourages calcium mobilization from bones. However, this function has negligible value in cattle because they excrete only small amounts of phosphate in their urine except when they suffer from another metabolic disorder known as acidosis. All ruminants commonly have alkaline urine and if they excreted mineral in their urine it would tend to precipitate (see Chapter 3, p. 41).

The point to emphasize is that parathyroid hormone stimulates calcium mobilization but takes several hours to accomplish the task. Thus, parathyroid hormone acts in the long-term control of calcium homeostasis leaving short-term adjustments to another hormone known as calcitonin.

Calcitonin works in the reverse mode to that of parathyroid hormone. It decreases calcium concentration in the blood. It is synthesized in, and secreted from, the so-called C-cells of the thyroid gland in response to hypercalcaemia. Even small rises in blood calcium provoke a rapid increase in blood calcitonin and a correspondingly rapid reduction in calcium levels. It works mainly by the suppression of bone resorption. It also promotes phosphate resorption from the urine by the kidneys—of negligible value in the ruminant as explained above.

The function of vitamin D_3 as a hormone only recently came to the fore. As cholecalciferol it enters the body from the food or by synthesis in the skin under the influence of ultraviolet irradiation from sunlight. However, cholecalciferol as such possesses little physiological activity needing first to be hydroxylated in two stages. The first hydroxylation involves conversion to 25-hydroxy-cholecalciferol in the liver, a process which is virtually uncontrolled. The second conversion to 1,25-dihydroxychole-calciferol occurs in the kidney under stimulation from parathyroid hormone. This fully hydroxylated compound then promotes the synthesis of calcium-binding protein and thus increases calcium absorption via the intestinal mucosa. The point to emphasize is that vitamin D_3 and parathyroid hormone work together in promoting the input of calcium.

Input/output relationships

Calcium

The calcium within a cow's body amounts to about 6 kg. Nearly all of this (88%) is stored in the skeleton where among other functions it serves as a reserve for the very small but vital proportion (1%) circulating in body fluids and soft tissues. In fact, the total calcium in the blood amounts to only about 8 g though the immediately available pool of calcium circulating in all body fluids is somewhat larger at about 16 g. The knife edge on which calcium metabolism in the cow is poised comes into focus when it is realized that a day's yield of say 30 kg milk (1.2 g Ca/kg), contains 36 g calcium representing over four times the calcium in the blood. It must replace its blood calcium very fast to cope with the demand for milk production and avoid hypocalcaemia. Any interference with intestinal absorption or with bone resorption could be rapidly fatal. This is particularly prone to happen at parturition when the calcium demands of the newly lactating udder must be met and metabolism must adjust rapidly just at a time when bouts of alimentary stasis commonly occur.

Disagreement exists on the nutritional standards for the calcium intake of the dairy cow. Feeding trials give conflicting assessments because variation in availability by absorption from the gut means that the actual intake commonly differs from that intended. Low availability leads to a variety of metabolic disorders, even on an apparently adequate diet.

Variation in absorption of calcium stems from several factors. Age is the most important because although calcium availability approaches 100% in calves on a liquid milk diet, with advancing age and maturity the availability falls to below 50% and even lower in old age. Much depends on the animals need for calcium. Absorption increases with need and especially in lactation—in other words, cows tend to absorb what they need but no more. Thus as dietary intake rises absorption falls. Doubling or trebling intake merely results in a downward adjustment of intake so that the net amount absorbed returns to the same constant value after a few days. There is thus no point in increasing dietary intake when need is satisfied because the excess passes out unabsorbed into the faeces.

Other factors affect absorption. The calcium : phosphorus ratio in the diet is an example. It reaches an optimal level at about 2:1. Cows tolerate wide departures from this with little harm at 4:1 or even 7:1, though at this level of imbalance the possibility of phosphorus deficiency needs attention. A practical problem related to this is that many cows receive unavoidably high intakes of calcium as, for instance, on chalk downland pasture so that a reasonable Ca:P ratio may be impossible to achieve. As will be seen later, the practical formulation of diets low in calcium for the prevention of parturient paresis is difficult.

Vitamin D exerts an effect and is vital for calcium absorption. However, supplements above actual need promote excess absorption and may even induce calcification of soft tissues. Protein intake also affects calcium absorption. Low protein diets interfere with absorption and skeletal development so that an ample intake of protein is vital to prevent bone pathology. Finally, excessive intake of magnesium reduces calcium absorption—possibly because magnesium competes with calcium for a common pathway through the gut mucosa.

It is generally agreed that nearly all cows undergo negative calcium balance during early lactation. Many consider this normal and even inevitable. Some estimates show that as much as 18% of skeletal mineral may be lost in one lactation but this is of little consequence in the long term if the reserves are replaced during the dry period.

Mineral interchange into and out of the bones occurs throughout life, though its importance in young animals to provide for their growth ranks high. With advancing age this interchange declines substantially. Thus the skeletal reserves become less labile and relatively unavailable for the older cow, which is one reason why such animals are prone to parturient hypocalcaemia.

Two other factors contribute to lability of bone metabolism. Relatively acidic diets (excess non-metabolizable anions) seem to increase the availability of calcium whereas relatively alkaline diets (excess non-metabolizable cations) work in reverse. Also, diets relatively deficient in magnesium suppress calcium availability. Both factors have relevance to parturient hypocalcaemia.

Finally, the endogenous loss of calcium via the digestive secretions and into the faeces needs mention. Estimates using radioisotopes put this at about 8–9 g/day, but the important point is that this loss is irreversible. Even on deficient diets endogenous output still continues so that cumulative losses gradually deplete reserves and eventually lead to bone pathology.

Phosphorus

The phosphorus content of a mature cow amounts to about 2.8 kg, i.e. about half that of calcium. It is also distributed differently. The Ca : P ratio in bone is 2 : 1. Thus there is about half the amount of phosphorus in the skeleton as compared with that of calcium, but relatively more phosphorus occurs in the body fluids and soft tissues. The concentration of phosphorus in muscle is 2–3 g P/kg compared with 0.1 g Ca/kg. Thus phosphorus deficiency leads rapidly to ill-thrift and poor growth, whereas calcium deficiency may remain unnoticed for a long time until it results eventually in bone disorder. Phosphorus has many physiological functions unrelated to those of calcium. It is a component of nucleoprotein and hence a vital factor in tissue growth. It is involved in metabolic pathways such as the transport of phospholipids. Several nutrients are absorbed from the gut in phosphorylated forms and it is a component of energy-rich compounds such as ATP and creatine phosphate. These functions clearly emphasize why phosphorus deficient animals fail to thrive.

In ruminants the phosphorus content of saliva makes an important contribution to metabolism. Very large amounts are excreted daily in this way but most of the salivary phosphate is resorbed lower down the alimentary tract. Two points emerge. First, phosphorus homeostasis depends on the alimentary recycling of phosphorus through the saliva and then re-entering lower down the alimentary tract. Any interruption to this cycle soon leads to hypophosphataemia. Even in normal circumstances the endogenous loss of phosphorus in the digestive secretions and out into the faeces is large (10 g/day) and relatively more than that of calcium. Second, the phosphorus input into the rumen is vital to promote the activity of the ruminal flora and fauna. Without this the ruminant cannot thrive because it fails to digest its food.

The availability of phosphorus from dietary input varies and resembles that of calcium. It is high in calves—over 90%—but falls with maturity to 55%. Estimates of need vary. Standards dating from the 1950–1960 period suggested that high intakes of phosphorus were needed. A cow giving 30 kg milk/day was said to need 85 g, but this standard is now reduced to 60 g daily. Caution has been expressed about this reduction, but no real harm appears to have resulted in animals fed on the revised standard.

An overall view of calcium and phosphorus metabolism reveals an important problem of imbalance. Milk contains approximately 1.2 g Ca/kg and 1.0 g P/kg, a Ca:P ratio of nearly 1:1. However, optimal absorption from food needs a Ca:P ratio of 2:1 and bone also contains a Ca:P ratio of 2:1, indicating that in normal metabolism a relative deficiency of phosphorus is likely. Various factors tend to correct for this inbuilt problem. In particular, cereals usually contain ample phosphorus, and concentrate rations for cows are frequently based on a cereal component and most also have added mineral supplements. Thus cows receiving concentrates may avoid phosphorus deficiency. The real problem arises when attempts are made to produce milk from cows fed solely on pasture or conserved forage without adequate supplementation with concentrates.

Magnesium

The total magnesium in an adult cow amounts to about 200 g, 70% of which is locked in the skeleton where it is not easily recoverable. Soft tissues account for 29% but only 1% circulates in the body fluids. This small, immediately available reserve—only about 2 g— is vital for normal physiology and if magnesium concentration in the blood plasma drops below its normal value of 2.5 mg/100 ml to less than 1 mg/100 ml fatal hypomagnesaemia usually follows. Unfortunately, the input/output channels are poorly regulated; milk yield imposes an irreversible drain and absorption of magnesium from the gut reacts to variable interacting factors. Not surprisingly homeostasis commonly fails.

The input of magnesium into the metabolic system depends largely on the availability of dietary supplies. A simple state of deficiency explains hypomagnesaemia in calves and in cattle grazing poor pasture. Calves need over 5 g/day and, assuming 70% availability, with milk containing 0.15 g/kg, then at least 5.7 kg of milk is needed daily to avoid hypomagnesaemia. Not surprisingly magnesium deficiency occurs in milk-fed calves. Similarly, in the grazing cow, 26.4 g Mg/day is needed for 30 kg milk yield/day. This may not be forthcoming from all pastures.

However, the real problem leading to grass tetany arises because of variability in the availability of magnesium from pasture plants. Magnesium in dry roughage and concentrates is more available (10–40%) than from fresh young grass (5–33%). Young grass with a high content of protein and potassium inhibits magnesium absorption and contributes to the 'tetany prone potential' of young rapidly grown swards.

Bone metabolism is little involved in magnesium homeostasis. There seems to be no mechanism for withdrawing magnesium from bone to cope with deficiency. However, the kidneys play a vital role in preventing hypermagnesaemia. Excess magnesium spills over into the urine. Conversely, if plasma magnesium falls below normal, urine levels drop to practically nil. This spill-over mechanism not only works effectively in preventing hypermagnesaemia, but it also gives a useful diagnostic sign of magnesium adequacy.

Parturient hypocalcaemia

Introduction

Synonyms include parturient paresis and milk fever (though in fact the body temperature of the affected cow is usually subnormal). This is an acute metabolic disorder, a regular and diagnostic feature of which is hypocalcaemia, the blood plasma calcium falling rapidly from the normal 9.5 mg/dl to below 5 mg/dl. Paresis supervenes as the calcium concentration falls to this low level and the animal becomes comatose. Nearly all cases occur within 3 days of parturition.

Several factors affect incidence, age strongly so. The incidence rises from 0.2% at the 1st calving to 9.6% by the 6th and, depending on which survey is quoted, eventually to 18%.

Certain herds suffer more than others and incidences of over 25% are recorded. Predisposing factors may operate on a herd basis because 'outbreaks' occur in certain herds in some seasons. A genetic relationship also exists and some breeds are more susceptible than others. For instance, Channel Island cows suffer more commonly than Friesians or Ayrshires. The actual hereditability of incidence is said to be only 12.8% and, as might be expected, breeding for milk production correlates positively with rising incidence.

Relationship to parturition is clear—22% of cases occur just before calving, 60.7% within 1 day, 14.5% at 2 days after and 2.8% 3 days after. Seasonal incidence occurs, with most cases in September and October which coincides with the autumn calving period. Many point out that incidence rises year by year in line with increases in milk production per cow.

Historically, parturient hypocalcaemia has been known for a long time. The first identifiable recorded case is claimed for 1793—interestingly enough at a time when selection for high yield and intensive milk production began. Reports in the nineteenth century linked the disease to apoplexy and to infection of the uterus and udder. Copious bleeding and 'powerful' medicines of beer with alum and nitre were recommended. The Danish veterinarian

Jungens Schmidt brought in a modern view in 1897. Although he mistakenly thought the disease was due to an udder infection he discovered that intramammary infusion of potassium iodide solution dramatically effected cures. With this treatment mortality fell from 70% to 15%. Soon it was found that infusions of water or saline were just as good and simply inflating the udder with air even more so. The next breakthrough came in 1925 when Dryere and Grieg suggested that the disease was really a hypocalcaemia probably caused by the sudden drain of calcium into the newly lactating udder. Mistakenly at that time they blamed parathyroid gland deficiency as the cause. However, this erroneous view did not adversely affect the treatment. Parenteral injection of calcium solutions were highly effective and by 1935 a non-irritant, non-toxic preparation (calcium borogluconate) appeared on the market. This treatment has stood the test of over 50 years use and even at that early stage our knowledge seemed both sufficient and complete but, however effective the cure, it still did not prevent the disease and its incidence continuing to rise. Also the availability of an effective treatment did not prevent losses of cows which died before they could be injected.

The cause

The cause of parturient hypocalcaemia is complex. At its simplest it is a failure of calcium homeostasis at the beginning of lactation. The sudden need to provide calcium for the synthesis of colostrum in the newly lactating udder provides the major precipitating factor in this failure, but added to it is the complex sequence of stress and interactions imposed by parturition. In particular, disruption in the normal pattern of feeding and digestion at calving upsets the delicate balance of mineral metabolism.

What is the problem in quantitative terms? The fetal calf at term takes only about 0.2 g Ca/hour across the placenta. This ceases as soon as it is born, but is replaced by the much greater demand imposed by lactation which takes up over 1 g Ca/hour; in high-producing cows this may even approach 2 g Ca/hour. Most cows eventually adapt by adjusting the rates of inflow and outflow of calcium, but even so this adaptation is imperfect because transient hypocalcaemia is the rule involving a fall from the normal of 9.5 mg/dl down to 7.0 mg/dl, especially in older cows at their third, or subsequent calvings. The severity of the hypocalcaemia depends only in part on the output of calcium into the milk on the first day of lactation. However, the vital point is that some cows suffer a greater degree of hypocalcaemia than others even with the same milk output. A critical level of plasma calcium supervenes at 6.5 mg/dl, because this level of hypocalcaemia seems to be incompatible with alimentary motility. Then stasis of the gastrointestinal tract cuts off the supply of calcium from the food and the cows suffer a rapid and severe hypocalcaemia, down to about 4.5 mg/dl, at which point clinical signs arise.

Much depends on the rate at which cows adapt to the extra need for calcium immediately after parturition. Assuming 30 litres of blood circulating in a typical cow, then this contains 8 g of calcium. The cow can afford to lose less than half of this before it reaches the danger point of collapse and this represents only one-sixth of the calcium needed in the first day's lactation. The situation is fundamentally unstable. We know experimentally (using infusions of calcium chelating agent EDTA) that only a few cows can mobilize an extra 0.8 g Ca/hour even in favourable circumstances, but estimates show that in late pregnancy this rate is even reduced to only 0.4 g Ca/hour. So how do cows normally adjust, because not all of them succumb? Experimentally, the process of adjustment has proved difficult to measure over the short time scale of parturition. However, the emergency mechanism seems to involve a temporary decrease in the major outflows of calcium to form new bone or to be secreted endogenously into the faeces. Longer-term adjustment depends on increased absorption of calcium from the alimentary tract. Still later there is an increasing tendency for extra calcium to be removed from bone.

Various factors adversely affect the adaptation and determine whether or not an individual cow proceeds to become a clinical case. First, milk yield ranks as the most important. Beef cows with low yields rarely succumb and cows with udders experimentally removed do not show even the normal degree of hypocalcaemia at calving. However, by no means all high-yielding cows get parturient hypocalcaemia. Hence milk yield, though important, cannot be the only factor.

Second, advancing age imposes a general slowing down of metabolism. The interchange of mineral in bone in older cows declines and so does the capacity of the gut to absorb calcium. In addition the rate at which ingesta passes through the alimentary tract slows down. All these changes inevitably impair the capacity of adjustment to extra demand. Thus older cows are more at risk and this fits the clinical situation.

The third predisposing factor concerns the dietary calcium intake before calving. Cows receiving excess are much more susceptible than those receiving comparatively little. This well-established factor suggests that a hormonal mechanism may be involved; indeed, the possible importance of parathyroid dysfunction seemed at first sight to be an attractive possibility. However, parathyroid response to hypocalcaemia is just as vigorous in milk fever-prone cows as in others. There is no lack of parathyroid hormone in clinical cases of hypocalcaemia and the injection of more parathyroid hormone has no value. Parathyroidectomized cows may even calve quite normally without suffering from parturient paresis.

This does not rule out an alternative hormonal theory for explaining susceptibility. Excess calcium intake may stimulate the thyroid C-cells to secrete calcitonin. Calcitonin is active in dairy cows on a day to day basis because most cows consume too much calcium. Also, intravenous injections of extra calcitonin provoke severe hypocalcaemia even to the point of clinical signs. Thus high-calcium diets might prime the mineral metabolism to come under the influence of calcitonin, thus alerting those systems which lead towards hypocalcaemia whilst inhibiting those capable of mobilizing extra supplies. Clinicians may feel that the importance of calcitonin in milk fever susceptibility remains merely an academic matter but the answer to many outbreaks of milk fever is simply to adjust mineral balance towards low calcium status during late pregnancy (see Prevention, p. 23).

The fourth predisposing factor is alimentary stasis. The lactating dairy cow depends on the continuous functioning of its alimentary tract and even brief interruption can lead to clinical hypocalcaemia. This has been induced experimentally by hyoscine and hypocalcaemic paresis ensued within 2 hours. Similar periods of stasis commonly occur at parturition. It is also pointed out above that hypocalcaemia itself induces and maintains alimentary stasis so that once the syndrome starts it enters a vicious circle, only relieved by treatment with calcium borogluconate to raise the blood calcium levels.

Some types of feed predispose to stasis, especially lush autumn grass and diets containing highly digestible concentrates and silage. In contrast, roughages such as hay and even barley straw are said to be beneficial in maintaining alimentary function.

Certain hormonal interactions cause alimentary stasis. For example, cows come under oestrogen stimulation at calving, which is known to induce inappetance and rapid declines in plasma ultrafilterable calcium. However, cows susceptible to milk fever seem to be no different from others in oestrogen status. The possibility remains that an oestrogen effect might just tip the balance at parturition and it certainly explains the occasional case of milk fever that occurs later in lactation coincident with oestrus.

Finally, certain dietary imbalances predispose to parturient hypocalcaemia. An example is the relative 'acidity' or 'alkalinity' of the total diet. These terms refer to the proportions of non-metabolizable cations to anions. For instance, sodium bicarbonate is composed of a non-metabolizable cation, sodium, and the metabolizable anion, bicarbonate. If the diet contains a relative excess of non-metabolizable anions, whether of calcium, magnesium, potassium or sodium there appears to be a reduction in the mobilizable reserves of calcium. On the other hand, relatively 'acidic' diets are said to be prophylactic for milk fever and the addition of ammonium chloride supplement is sometimes beneficial.

Another important dietary imbalance causing milk fever is magnesium deficiency. This has special importance in 'outbreaks' of the disorder that occur on autumn pasture. Experimentally, even very mild deficiency of magnesium with hypomagnesaemia inhibits the mobilization of calcium presumably by a direct effect on bone metabolism. On the other hand, excessive intakes of magnesium may also provoke parturient hypocalcaemia. Thus over-zealous preventive measures against hypomagnesaemia may end up with the reverse effect of that intended. Excess magnesium is thought to interfere with calcium absorption from the gut and may even stimulate calcitonin secretion, which would in turn bring on a reduction in blood calcium.

Clinical signs and diagnosis

Hypocalcaemia, the characteristic and diagnostic feature of the disorder, is the basis for the clinical signs. Low concentrations of blood calcium lead initially to hypersensitivity of the conducting membranes in nerves and muscles and then to hyperexcitability and tetany. In the later stages of parturient paresis, however, contrary to expectation, muscle paralysis and not tetany is the rule. The suggested explanation is that the hypocalcaemia increases cell permeability to cations and thus potassium leaks out of the cell and sodium enters. This reduces the potential difference across the cell membrane which paralyses muscle contractions. In turn this brings on another undesirable event. Increased permeability of cells allows phosphate to leak out, thus leading to degeneration and necrosis of muscle fibres. This could predispose to the 'downer-cow' syndrome in which cows fail to rise even though treated with calcium borogluconate.

Parturient paresis occurs so commonly within the narrow time limit of 3 days after parturition that almost any recumbent newly-calved cow is assumed to be suffering from it. Satisfactory response to calcium borogluconate treatment merely adds confirmation. However, differential diagnosis is important. The first complicating factor is that various types of injury, including ruptured tendons, fractured bones and torn muscles also cause recumbency. Fortunately, the clinical signs of parturient paresis are so characteristic that blood analysis is rarely called upon for confirmation. Should this be necessary all genuine cases of parturient paresis have blood plasma or serum calcium well below 7 mg/dl, and usually below 5 mg/dl. In a simple case this is usually accompanied by hypophosphataemia and hyperglycaemia.

Differential diagnosis must also take into account the so-called complex forms of parturient paresis. Each may need a specially designed approach to treatment and prevention. Serum magnesium, though commonly high in simple cases, can sometimes be low—this occurs in those 'outbreaks' of milk fever described above where low magnesium status is a susceptibility factor. Such complex cases, involving both hypomagnesaemia and hypocalcaemia, show more hyperexcitability than simple cases, especially before severe signs commence, and are difficult to treat. Even greater complexity is introduced when hypoglycaemia occurs as well. In these circumstances a starvation syndrome supervenes with a very difficult combination of parturient hypocalcaemia, grass tetany and ketosis. Such cases commonly occur on lush, though poor quality, autumn pasture, and even though the animals may appear to be in good condition fatty liver is often found to be yet another complication.

Cows succumbing to parturient hypocalcaemia commonly go through a sequence of stages. The first is so brief it may not be seen. Hyperexcitement and hypersensitivity comes on with muscle tremors, twitching, drooping ears, etc. The hind legs stiffen and the cow may 'paddle' from side to side. Soon she falls stiffly to the ground, often into an uncomfortable position or in an awkward place (for example, a pond or stream or narrow corridor). The second stage involves sternal recumbency. The cow becomes depressed and almost unconscious. She cannot rise and turns her muzzle into her flank. Hypothermia begins. Ruminal stasis and constipation become apparent. The third stage involves complete collapse and coma. The cardiovascular system now fails as shown by a weak pulse and heart sounds; this can create a practical problem in raising the jugular vein for intravenous therapy. Within a few hours of this the cow dies unless treated—in fact, before a satisfactory method was discovered about 90% of such cases had a fatal outcome. A common cause of death is respiratory failure from bloat, but cardiovascular collapse commonly occurs terminally.

Prevention and treatment

Prevention

The strategy for prevention depends on the situation operative on the actual farm. A low and sporadic incidence of only 5% is too low to repay the cost of preventive measures unless especially susceptible groups of cows can be identified to simplify the effort. For example, some cows undergo milk fever at successive calvings, or belong to susceptible family lines. They deserve individual attention, possibly by means of massive injections of vitamin D_3 (10 million IU).

Vigorous preventive measures apply in herds with a known high incidence, or when 'outbreaks' occur. The first step means choosing the right strategy because some methods fail if applied in the wrong circumstances. For instance, prophylaxis with vitamin D_3 will not work when the background factor is chronic hypomagnesaemia. The decision for each herd depends on the answers to the following questions.

relapses tend to occur, and that 12 g is too much. Intravenous calcium in these quantities raises blood calcium well above normal and induces irregularities in heart beat which can be detected readily. However, acute toxicity with calcium borogluconate is low because the calcium cation is bound to the borogluconate anion and thus kept in a temporarily inactive form.

Calcium borogluconate is the standard treatment but should a complex type of parturient paresis be suspected, then solutions containing magnesium and/or dextrose additions can be used to advantage.

Trials indicate that a double injection of calcium borogluconate given both intravenously and subcutaneously gives advantage. The intravenous calcium gives immediate effect whilst a depot beneath the skin gives slower but longer cover.

Most animals recover rapidly after treatment. Within 5–10 minutes the cow's head rises, she passes faeces and attempts to get up. If relapse occurs it commonly happens within 24 hours and needs a second treatment; for some unfortunate cows this cycle of cure and relapse may repeat itself until the mineral metabolism eventually adjusts. Repeated relapses can be stopped if necessary by inflation of the udder with air to inhibit further secretion and loss of calcium into the milk.

Failure to rise after 12 hours indicates the need for re-treatment but blood tests can check if the delay in recovery follows from genuine hypocalcaemia, or from another cause such as muscle damage. Enforced recumbency always inflicts damage due to pressure restriction of blood supply to the muscles. Thus treatment should always include nursing to raise the cow onto her brisket and to turn her from side to side at hourly intervals. A recumbent cow always needs frequent observation and good nursing if she is to recover effectively and completely.

The downer cow

Recumbent cows, failing to rise after an otherwise successful treatment for parturient paresis, are called 'downer cows'. They seem alert but unable to stand, apparently because of hindleg paralysis. Some can get up onto their forelimbs and crawl forwards dragging their hindquarters behind—these are commonly called 'creepers'. The whole syndrome of the downer cow is not a separate and distinct metabolic disorder, but merely an unfortunate sequel to parturient paresis.

The cause in most cases follows from pressure necrosis of the muscle and nerves of the hind limb. Even 4–6 hours recumbency is enough to induce ischaemic myonecrosis and neuropathology, especially if the cow falls onto its side directly upon a hard concrete floor. The extent of the resultant damage governs the likely prognosis and chances of eventual recovery. This can be gauged by a blood enzyme profile. Serum glutamic oxalo transaminase (GOT) and creatine phosphokinase (CPK) probably find most favour because these enzymes leak from damaged muscle fibres and the degree of increase in their concentrations in the blood correlates with the extent of the muscle damage and with the probability of recovery. In severe cases myohaemoglobin can be detected in the blood and urine. In fact, many consider that much increased levels of serum GOT and/or a strongly positive myoglobin reaction in the urine indicates such severe disintegration of tissue that recovery is unlikely.

Several causes of recumbency occur apart from pressure necrosis of muscle. For instance, incoordinated attempts to stand can inflict extensive tearing and haemorrhage in muscles especially if the cow spread-eagles across a slippery concrete floor. There may even be pelvic fractures caused by the impact of the falling cow during her initial collapse. The main sciatic nerve may be damaged and there may be obturator paralysis caused by the trauma of parturition. Finally, the cow may suffer from another coincidental and incapacitating disease such as mastitis or metritis, or she may simply be exhausted after a long and difficult calving. Whatever the cause the eventual outcome is always in doubt. In general, recumbency for up to a week is still compatible with complete recovery, but it rarely follows after a 2 week involvement.

The downer cow seldom shows clinical signs of parturient hypocalcaemia. The blood levels of calcium, phosphorus, magnesium and glucose are usually within the normal range. If not, then intravenous therapy with an appropriate mixture may help recovery. However, care is needed. Repeated injections of calcium can inflict myocardial damage. Some clinicians claim a good response to phosphate injection for the downer cow, feeling that leakage of phosphate from the muscle cells causes the degeneration. However, this hypothesis has not yet received full scientific support.

Treatment for the downer cow consists of careful nursing. Prompt movement of affected animals onto soft bedding prevents further damage and then they will need regular turning every 2–4 hours. Hind limbs must be massaged and frequent extension and flexion is necessary. Animals sometimes stay immobile for up to 7 days and even then make valiant attempts to rise. At this stage they may benefit from assistance using the various slings and tackle supports that are available, but great care is needed to prevent the infliction of even more trauma and muscle damage. Perhaps the best treatment for the downer cow is to exercise enough care and patience.

Grass tetany

Introduction

Synonyms include lactation tetany, acute hypomagnesaemia, hypomagnesaemic tetany and grass staggers. This is a highly fatal disease of ruminants, frequently so rapid in onset that clinical signs fail to be seen before the animals are found dead where they have fallen in the field. Grass tetany is especially liable to occur in cows grazing improved pasture and they seem to be most susceptible when lactating. The main diagnostic feature is hypomagnesaemia with the concentration of magnesium in the blood falling from the normal of 2.5 mg/dl to below 0.5 mg/dl. Care is needed in interpreting blood chemistry because many cows develop severe hypomagnesaemia without clinical signs. However, even these probably sit on the verge of collapse; the slightest stress might precipitate violent hyperexcitement and tetany. Most clinicians regard hypomagnesaemia in apparently normal cows as an important premonitory warning.

Hypomagnesaemic cows commonly show a concurrent hypocalcaemia which may be important clinically because the onset of tetany is said to be triggered by a sudden fall in serum calcium. Even a short period of fasting or stress may be enough to induce the hypocalcaemia and examples of such situations include transport, movement from field to field, sudden change in diet, transient indigestion, etc.

Although the incidence of grass tetany is generally low it frequently varies considerably between areas, herds and even between individual fields. An incidence of up to 2% is common, but catastrophic outbreaks, even involving up to 20%, occur on certain farms. Mortality of affected animals tends to be high and thus the economic cost of the disorder approaches that of milk fever which, although having a higher incidence, rarely kills before effective treatment is given. Fortunately, much is known about preventing grass tetany and thus the loss can be reduced considerably. In fact, it pays to put more effort into prevention, especially at times of greatest risk, so that treatment is seldom needed.

Grass tetany, unlike milk fever, is not normally related to parturition. However, lactating cows are especially susceptible because the demand for magnesium in the synthesis of milk imposes an additional burden on magnesium homeostasis. Also there is a pronounced seasonal trend, with most cases occurring when cattle go out from winter housing and feeding onto lush pasture in early spring. Another peak in incidence occurs in the autumn when cows rely on the low nutritional value of pasture at the tail end of the summer grazing. Particularly dangerous are those swards which have received generous nitrogen and potassium fertilization during the preceding months.

Historically, grass tetany has been known for a long time. The key discovery that its immediate cause was hypomagnesaemia coincided with similar reports that hypocalcaemia caused milk fever. The treatment proposed thus followed logically for both— parenteral calcium solutions worked well for milk fever and, in the same way, magnesium solutions seemed relatively effective for grass tetany. Realization soon followed that the condition was really a nutritional deficiency of magnesium conditioned by factors such as high intakes of potassium. The remaining difficulty was to formulate an effective preventive method involving magnesium supplementation of cattle under grazing conditions.

The cause

The cause of grass tetany is simply a failure of magnesium homeostasis in grazing ruminants. Housed animals fed concentrate rations and conserved forage are only rarely affected. Lactation imposes an additional demand for magnesium which explains why lactating cows seem to be especially at risk. The principal problem is inadequate intake of dietary magnesium coupled with certain factors which limit the absorption of magnesium from the intestine.

The problem can be viewed quantitatively. Milking cows theoretically need only about 20 g of magnesium daily to satisfy their needs. Unfortunately the absorption of magnesium varies; magnesium in lush grass is less available than that in dry conserved forage. Even the calcined magnesite currently used for supplementation may be poorly absorbed. Thus a simple computation of the magnesium content of the diet may mislead. Adding to the problem is the unfortunate fact that the reserves of magnesium locked away in the skeleton seem almost unavailable when needed. An important point to emphasize is that magnesium homeostasis has no firm endocrinological control like that of calcium and thus the animal depends on a regular intake of dietary magnesium to maintain blood magnesium concentration. As a general rule once magnesium in pasture herbage falls below 0.2% of dry matter then hypomagnesaemia becomes likely.

The situation is made complex by the following factors:

1 Young grass contains less available magnesium than mature or conserved grass.

2 Swards of monoculture ryegrass are low in magnesium content unlike clovers and other broad leaf plants.

3 Fertilization of the pasture with nitrogen and potassium inhibits the uptake of magnesium into the herbage and also prevents the absorption of magnesium across the intestinal mucosa.

4 Excessive dietary calcium appears to inhibit magnesium absorption and hence liming of pasture may increase its tetany potential for grazing livestock.

5 Proteinaceous feed which increases the ammonia content of the rumen inhibits magnesium absorption, possibly by the precipitation of magnesium ammonium phosphate.

6 Various magnesium chelating agents exist. These include ketobutyric acid, citrate or transaconitic acid. Although not of primary importance such chelating agents might convert an already critical situation into a clinical outbreak.

Clinical signs and diagnosis

Most cases progress so rapidly through severe clinical signs to death that no time remains for the stockman to pick out affected animals for treatment. The cow is just found dead where it collapsed in tetany. Careful observation usually reveals affected cows which suddenly bellow for no obvious reason in the middle of normal grazing. They often gallop off in frenzy and then fall in convulsions. Temporary recovery if it occurs may be followed by more convulsions and then death. Chronic cases do occur. In these the cow becomes obviously disturbed, she fails to eat and seems hypersensitive. She is awkward and even dangerous to handle and may continue so for several days before going on to the convulsion stage. Sometimes a whole herd behaves in this strange way though only a few progress to severe clinical signs and death. Many recover uneventfully.

Other signs of an acute case include hyperthermia, probably on account of the severe muscle contractions associated with tetany. Also the heart beats become irregular and so loud that they can be heard even at a distance.

Grass tetany may occur as a complication of parturient paresis. This is particularly likely in the autumn when all the cows in a herd may become hypomagnesaemic and hyperexcitable before calving. The hyperaesthesia and tetanic spasms become a feature of the paresis, distinguishable from the dull and flaccid collapse characteristic of typical parturient paresis.

Diagnosis usually depends on observing the clinical signs. However, the analysis of blood samples for hypomagnesaemia and hypocalcaemia adds confirmation. The regular monitoring of magnesium status in herd profile tests allows the detection of an impending problem so that preventive measures can be put in hand at an early preclinical stage.

Prevention and treatment

Prevention means increasing the intake of magnesium. Though this is simple, theoretically, practical problems remain. The usual method is to feed a magnesium supplement to give cover over the danger periods of turnout onto spring pasture or of grazing lush but nutritionally inadequate grass in late autumn. Calcined magnesite (MgO) in oral doses of 60 g daily usually protects, but this compound is poorly absorbed and may not always be sufficiently effective. Larger doses of up to 200 g daily can even be contraindicated because it interferes with calcium absorption and also causes scouring. The calcined magnesite can be given by drench, but it is more usual to incorporate the required amount into a supplementary feed if the cattle can be persuaded to eat it. Mixing with molasses often overcomes the problem. A soluble salt such as magnesium acetate in molasses given in a ball feeder works well, if expensively. Dusting the herbage with MgO at 125 kg/ha gives good protection but only temporarily, depending on how soon the rain washes the dust from the leaves. Top dressing with MgO at the higher level of 1125 kg/ha gives a greater and more permanent boost to pasture magnesium (up to 3 years on light soils). Although expensive, this treatment is more permanent and can be applied to a limited area for grazing during the periods of highest risk.

Magnesium alloy 'bullets' which allow the slow release of their contained magnesium, as they slowly dissolve in the rumen, tend to be relatively ineffective in maintaining blood magnesium because the amount released is slight compared with the cow's nutritional needs. However, they are said to give immediate cover in times of hypomagnesaemic crisis.

Other considerations need attention. First, much can be achieved by limiting the application of potassium fertilizers. Second, the danger of certain pastures recedes if the sward contains a proportion of legumes such as clover. Access to weeds in hedgerows or strips around the headlands can be beneficial. Third, careful management of the cattle is needed. Giving access to hay or rough grazing may assist the digestion and thus prevent interruption to the absorption of magnesium and, finally, the avoidance of stress can prevent a grass tetany outbreak in herds where the animals are already in a critical hypomagnesaemic state.

Treatment is urgently needed for affected animals. An intravenous injection of a combination of magnesium and calcium salts is usual but must be given slowly to avoid a fatal action on the heart. Some prefer to give the calcium solution intravenously but reserve the magnesium for subcutaneous use. Whichever route is chosen recovery may be good, but blood magnesium tends to fall back again within 24 hours and the clinical signs may recur.

Hypomagnesaemic tetany in calves

This condition resembles grass tetany in adult cattle and can be traced to low magnesium intake. The diets of milk-fed calves are deficient in magnesium with the result that such animals suffer chronic hypomagnesaemia. The low magnesium status resulting from milk diets may be exacerbated by the high calcium content of milk which inhibits magnesium absorption. Other factors which increase the danger include diarrhoea and the chewing of bedding both of which encourage the output of magnesium in the faeces or the saliva.

Housed calves are particularly affected. Frequently all the animals in a shed may become hyperexcitable and some will undergo tetany and die in convulsions.

Response to magnesium sulphate intravenously gives temporary relief, but dietary supplements with magnesium oxide or carbonate are advisable.

Bone disorders associated with inadequate or excess mineralization

Osteodystrophy finds increasing use as a general term describing disorders of bone involving either demineralization in adults or restriction of normal development in the young. Many types of bone disorder occur in cattle. Most involve nutritional inadequacy of either minerals or vitamins, which may involve an excess or imbalance of calcium, phosphorus or vitamin D, though other factors can play a secondary role. For instance, an apparent deficiency of phosphorus may fail to respond to appropriate supplementation because of an associated deficiency of protein or because the phosphorus supplement contains enough fluorine to induce fluorosis and its associated bone pathology. Also, even apparently well-fed lactating dairy cattle easily fall prey to bone disorder. Repeated pregnancy and lactation deplete their skeletal reserve and they gradually succumb to 'milk lameness'.

Bone disorders are not confined to deficient mineralization. In some cases bones over-calcify as in osteopetrosis. Finally, congenital disorders of bone occur, often leading to bizarre pathology of bone structure and function.

'Milk lameness' or osteoporosis

This is probably the commonest form of bone disorder in dairy cows. It is associated with the extreme output of mineral into the milk in high-yielding cows coupled with imbalances of their dietary input.

The cause

'Milk lameness' in dairy cattle is a typical production disease being due to imbalance between input and output. Much depends on the circumstances applicable on the farm concerned. If the feed consists mainly of roughage, produced on the farm itself with all its innate deficiencies, all continues well provided it is supplemented by an appropriately balanced concentrate feed. Problems arise when undue reliance rests solely on the pasture and locally grown roughage. For instance, chalk downland is deficient in phosphorus, though containing vast excess of calcium. On the other hand, soils overlying granite rocks tend towards acidity and calcium deficiency. Fortunately, cattle tolerate minor errors in input and suffer badly only when these are combined with high output, either in the form of rapid growth or copious lactation, which impose extra strain on the metabolism.

Phosphorus deficiency poses an especial problem for cattle. Not only is phosphorus a vital component of bone but it also provides an essential aid for digestion. In the saliva it acts as a buffer to preserve the optimum pH in the ruminal fluid and furthermore it provides a source of phosphorus for the growth of the ruminal flora and fauna. Thus phosphorus deficiency, although affecting bone metabolism directly, also imposes an added burden by limiting the proper digestion of nutrients essential for growth, such as protein. Bone metabolism depends on good protein status.

The molecular structure of bone bears directly on its susceptibility to disorder. Much of its solidity relies on minute crystals of a compound resembling hydroxyapatite [$Ca_{10} (PO_4)_6 (OH)_2$]. This has a calcium : phosphorus ratio of 2:1, whereas milk has a Ca : P ratio of nearly 1 : 1 and dietary intake is usually in excess of 3:1. These discrepancies mean that phosphorus requirements for lactation are at a premium and that the preservation of homeostasis may entail excessive mobilization of bone with the eventual outcome of bone pathology.

Newly formed bone contains a high proportion of amorphous calcium phosphate which crystallizes later. This interim material has value in presenting a very large surface area for rapid interchange. Not only does it serve as an immediately available reserve but it also sequestrates toxic elements such as lead and fluorine. Unfortunately, this potentially useful function carries a hazard because some of the sequestered material may induce bone pathology.

This applies particularly to fluorine because zealous attempts to correct 'milk lameness' with a phosphorus supplement may be frustrated if the supplement contains even very small amounts of fluorine. Such a supplement successfully stimulates the growth of new bone but this in turn possesses enhanced ability to absorb fluorine so that apparently subtoxic levels may still provoke clinical signs.

One of the main problems with a bone disorder such as 'milk lameness' is that it is a chronic, long-term condition. It is insidious in development. Minor imbalances persisting over many years gradually build up to a critical point in which several cows simultaneously show clinical signs. The mineral composition of the diet at this time many not be suspect but it fails to reflect the long-term imbalance. Furthermore, expert opinion on correct mineral status has varied over the years—intakes considered acceptable 20 years ago have changed more than once in the interim. Much of the discrepancy stems from lack of knowledge about the availability of minerals for absorption. Poor availability leads to bone disorder even on apparently adequate diets.

Availability depends on several interacting factors. Age is most important because calcium availability in calves approaches 100% and phosphorus 90%, but these values fall to less than 45% and 55% respectively with maturity. Adult cows tend to absorb calcium up to their needs but then no more—doubling or tripling the intake merely gives commensurate falls in absorption—the excess passing on unabsorbed into the faeces. As age advances availability falls even lower.

The calcium : phosphorus ratio in the diet affects availability. A ratio of 2:1 seems optimal, but below 1:1 or above 4:1 it becomes progressively less favourable. Ratios below 1:1 seem poorly tolerated but are not unusual in housed beef animals kept almost exclusively on cereal-based diets. In contrast, ratios of over 4:1

commonly occur on chalk downland and pasture. These are common for many highly-producing dairy herds. Also certain supplements seem less available than others.

Excess magnesium reduces both calcium and phosphorus availability. Magnesium seems to compete with calcium for absorption in a common pathway and also may combine with phosphorus to form relatively insoluble salts such as magnesium ammonium phosphate.

The type of food has an effect. Availability of calcium is low in most roughages but higher with cereals and in most concentrate rations.

A negative balance (excess output over input) for minerals is not unusual during lactation. Many query the practical importance of this, pointing out that reserves are replenished rapidly during the dry period. However, skeletal mineral commonly falls by up to 18% in one lactation which amounts to a considerable deficit to restore. This emphasizes the importance of proper mineral nutrition during the dry period and the need for adequate vitamin D intake to support mineral absorption and exchange in bone. Mention must be made at this point of the possible antagonistic effects of vitamin A to vitamin D because grazing cows take in a relative excess of its precursor, carotene. This could be yet another factor depressing calcium availability (see Chapter 9, p. 111).

In summary, the following causes of 'milk lameness' or osteoporosis occur in cattle:

1 Absolute deficiencies of calcium, phosphorus or vitamin D or wide imbalances in their proportions.

2 High output in the milk relative to input.

3 Interaction with other minerals such as magnesium.

4 Factors affecting availability.

Clinical signs and diagnosis

Defective mineralization of bone provokes very obvious clinical signs as shown by the names given to it in various countries. For example, these include cruban (Scotland), pegleg (Australia), boglame (Ireland) and stiffs (Florida). These names describe the inevitable results of weakening of the bone structure as it becomes denuded of mineral. The bones bend easily and distort even under normal weightbearing stress. They commonly undergo sponta-

neous fracture. Pain is felt and this in turn restricts grazing ability
and food intake. Long bones become bowed and swelling occurs at
their epiphyseal ends leading to stiff joints and lameness. Deleterious effects on the teeth include delay and irregularity in the
eruption of incisors with excessive wear of the molars.

Associated clinical signs include pica and infertility, especially
in phosphorus deficiency.

Blood chemistry provides a helpful diagnostic aid even before
clinical signs begin. Hypophosphataemia predicts low phosphorus
status and reference to hypoalbuminaemia may suggest low protein
status. Low concentrations of blood copper or caeruloplasmin also
indicate the possibility or otherwise of copper deficiency interacting in the pathogenesis of the bone disorder.

Prevention and treatment

Nutritional osteoporosis usually responds readily to appropriate
mineral supplementation provided time is allowed for the resol-
ution of long-standing lesions. Supplementation can be given
orally by simple addition to the diet but the benefit can be hastened
by parenteral vitamin D. In advanced cases additional supportive
therapy to ease the pain is indicated. This entails adequate bedding
and care when driving animals from pasture to milking parlours,
etc.

Rickets

Rickets occurs in growing calves and is due to defective mineralization of the developing bone. The cartilage of the growth plates at
the ends of the long bones fails to be resorbed and the bone matrix,
which is laid down in the rest of the bone substance, fails to be
calcified.

The cause

Rickets in calves is caused by a deficiency of vitamin D or phosphorus, or occasionally of calcium. Vitamin D deficiency tends to
occur in housed calves though pastured stock are more liable to
phosphorus deficiency in much the same way as are mature cows.
Rapid growth enhances the disorder. In these circumstances the

long bones attempt to elongate rapidly by the addition of cartilage at the epiphyses but this then fails to be resorbed or calcified. Growth in length ceases and the bones become so stunted and weak that they deform and bend under stress. The cartilaginous end plates, which remain unmineralized, tend to amass into thickened swellings around the joints. Calves on otherwise good diets suffer most because they grow the fastest.

Clinical signs and diagnosis

The affected calves become stiff and cannot walk properly. Their limb joints enlarge. Their ribs show nodular enlargements at the costochondrial junctions (the so-called 'ricketic rosary'). Seen from the front the limb bones are curved or bowed. The effect of rickets on the teeth can be most severe; not only is tooth eruption delayed but also defects in the jaws cause bad alignment of the teeth. The calves seem unable to close their mouths properly and have difficulty in feeding.

Diagnosis is generally straightforward, based on clinical signs coupled with an appraisal of dietary intake. Confirmatory evidence derives from blood chemistry. Serum inorganic phosphorus will be low and possibly also serum calcium—a rule of thumb guide is that clinical signs usually follow if the product of Ca × P falls below 30. A check on blood copper or caeruloplasmin helps distinguish rickets from the effects of copper deficiency (see Chapter 8, p. 95).

The appearance of the bones at post-mortem examination is characteristic; they are soft and demineralized with an ash content below 45% of their total weight. Radiographic evidence will seldom be needed for diagnosis in calves.

Prevention and treatment

Recovery usually follows the correction of the dietary deficiency, but residual and long-term lesions usually persist. Care in management may assist recovery.

Enzootic calcinosis

Enzootic calcinosis caused by poisoning with certain plants or by excess vitamin D and its analogues receives increasing recognition in various parts of the world. Similar, probably identical, disorders occur in Jamaica (Manchester wasting disease), Brazil (Espichamenta), Hawaii (Naalehy), Argentina (Enteque seco) as well as in West Germany (Enzootic calcinosis). The common feature is extensive calcification of soft tissue (metastatic calcification). A similar disorder follows massive doses of vitamin D_3 if used over-zealously for the prevention of milk fever.

Causes

Various plants contain poisons which possess toxins having intense vitamin D activity. In most cases the toxin involved seems to be a glycoside of 1α, 25-dihydroxycholecalciferol which acts in the body in the same way as vitamin D. However, its toxicity is especially potent because it needs no further hydroxylation for full activity. There is also some evidence that the effects of the poisoning are exacerbated by mineral imbalances in the soil and herbage. The plants involved include *Solanum malocoxylon* (Argentina), *Trisetum flavescens* (West Germany) and *Cestrum diurnum* (USA). Cattle consume these plants in various ways. For instance, *S. malocoxylon*, which grows in damp or wet soils, is rarely eaten by cattle except in dry periods when other plants cease to be available. In contrast, *T. flavescens* seems to be most toxic when the plant is young and green. Silage retains the toxic principle but it tends to be destroyed at haymaking

Ingestion of these plants induces hypercalcaemia and hyperphosphataemia, often over 20% above normal concentrations. Serum calcium may reach 13 mg/dl and inorganic phosphorus even up to 12 mg/dl. This is associated with a massive increase in mineral absorption from the diet. It seems certain that these effects are mediated by a metabolite of vitamin D_3 namely 1,25-dihydroxycholecalciferol.

Clinical signs and diagnosis

The incidence of the disorder varies (10–50% in affected areas), depending on how much of the plants are eaten. *S. malocoxylon* seems to be toxic in very small amounts but *T. flavescens* is less toxic. The disorder takes time to develop—even up to 1 year or more—but slowly progresses. Clinical signs include loss of appetite and wasting occurs accompanied by lameness and pain. Excessive thirst and urination is another feature. The heart and breathing become increasingly laboured so that the animals are progressively incapable of walking.

Mortality can attain 60% of affected cattle. At post-mortem examination calcified plaques, seen as white, gritty inclusions are observed throughout the body, but especially beneath the endothelial lining of the heart and arteries. The bones show osteopetrosis (excessive mineralization) and the kidneys contain calcified tubules with stones in the renal pelvis.

Diagnosis presents no problem especially in enzootic areas where the disease is well known. The clinical signs and post-mortem appearance are characteristic. Blood chemistry merely adds confirmation.

Prevention and treatment

Prevention depends on separating the animals from the toxic plant. However, once established the lesions rarely resolve. Treatment is not usually attempted, but aluminium hydroxide therapy has been tried in sheep.

Osteopetrosis

Alternative names include 'marble bone'. It occurs especially in bulls fed diets which contain high levels of minerals more suitable for lactating cows. A congenital form of osteopetrosis is said to occur in Aberdeen Angus calves in which the long bones are shortened with no marrow cavity.

The cause

The cause of osteopetrosis in bulls stems from an excessive intake of calcium and phosphorus. Bulls at stud commonly receive diets containing over 90 g Ca and 60 g P, which is well over actual needs. The excess calcium leads to temporary hypercalcaemia which in turn triggers a response from the thyroid C-cells to secrete calcitonin. If the situation of excess calcium status persists the thyroid

C-cells initially undergo hyperplasia which then progresses to neoplasia. Over 60% of bulls in some studs may show such effects.

The excess secretion of calcitonin successfully suppresses the hypercalcaemia but also inhibits bone resorption so that gradually the skeleton becomes abnormally calcified. The bones increase in density and produce outgrowths or osteophytes especially in the vertebrae, which may eventually fuse. Similar lesions may form adjacent to other joints.

Clinical signs and diagnosis

Affected bulls become lame, suffer pain and joint stiffness. Eventually they cannot serve or ejaculate and must be culled. Diagnosis depends on clinical signs and the presence of typical lesions at post-mortem examination.

Prevention and treatment

Treatment is not attempted. Prevention relies upon feeding appropriate diets for non-lactating animals such as bulls (see Chapter 9, p. 109 for the effect of vitamin A on the remodelling of bone).

3 / Urolithiasis

Urolithiasis means the formation of calculi in the urinary tract. It ranks as a metabolic disorder because it is mainly due to nutritional factors, which include excessive or imbalanced intakes of minerals. The calculi obstruct the urinary tract causing retention of the urine. The problem assumes special importance in castrated male steers in whom the penis and the urethra remain sexually under-developed and small, so that even small calculi tend to lodge. Urolithiasis not only causes important losses economically but it also inflicts severe suffering with pain, possible rupture of the bladder and death.

The cause

Several factors combine to make cattle prone to urolithiasis. Many of these depend on the chemical characteristics of their urine. Normal urine of cattle is alkaline because it contains large amounts of potassium bicarbonate, the potassium being eaten in herbage from the pasture. Unfortunately, at high pH calcium and phosphorus are relatively insoluble, which limits the amount of mineral which can be excreted safely without danger of precipitation. An additional hazard is that any excess magnesium absorbed from the alimentary tract passes out quantitatively via the kidneys. This magnesium forms complex insoluble salts with calcium and phosphorus should these be present.

It is important to determine the circumstances in which the urine of cattle changes from normal to containing sufficient concentrations of calcium, phosphorus or magnesium for calculi to form. One of these circumstances occurs in fattening cattle, which frequently receive cereal-based diets containing excess phosphorus and magnesium, but relatively low in calcium and potassium. Urinary pH falls, phosphate and magnesium concentrations rise and the urine supersaturates with mineral salts which precipitate into calculi. The composition of these calculi varies, but is commonly a complex mixture of calcium, magnesium and phosphate.

The incidence of calculi is highest in young male calves, especially those castrated early and fed a high grain diet with a calcium: phosphorus ratio as low as 1:1. In these circumstances the calculi are generally of the phosphatic type containing calcium, magnesium and ammonium phosphates.

Other forms of calculi occur. Cattle on pasture or fed indoors on plants containing large amounts of oxalate develop calculi due to the precipitation of calcium oxalate after excretion via the kidneys. Also, plants containing large amounts of silica have been associated with the danger of silicious calculi.

Urine is commonly a highly saturated solution of a variety of salts, many of which exceed their solubility products. The logical question is why calculi do not always occur. One theory is that urine contains a number of protective colloids which form a complex gel in which precipitation is inhibited. However, the important point remains that urine is an unstable solution and any one of a number of factors may combine to allow precipitation. Even normal urine contains some crystals in suspension, the quantity of which can be estimated using haematocrit tubes. A high concentration of crystals predicts impending urolithiasis.

Several factors interact in predisposing to calculi formation. The presence of a nidus composed of desquamated epithelial cells or other cellular debris may favour the deposition of insoluble salts around itself. Thus, urolithiasis is especially liable to occur in association with cystitis or nephritis when accumulation of pus or other debris gives ample provision of nidi.

As mentioned above, the pH of urine affects the solubility of some solutes. For instance, phosphate and carbonate calculi precipitate out more readily in an alkaline than in an acid medium. The relative concentration of salts in the urine is important especially in the precipitation of calculi containing silica. Cattle on pasture may consume and excrete large amounts of silica (as high as 6% from some plants), and this tends to precipitate when the animals drink only small amounts of water and the urine becomes concentrated. Yet another factor favouring the growth of calculi is associated with certain mucoproteins. These are said to be excreted in rapidly growing animals which have a rapid turnover of intercellular materials. The mucoprotein acts as a cement which enables the calculi to grow in concentric rings.

Finally, a very rare and specific type of urolithiasis occurs as an inherited problem. Affected cattle are deficient in xanthine oxidase and must excrete xanthine in their urine with the result that they become liable to xanthine calculi.

Clinical signs and diagnosis

Calculi do not commonly cause clinical signs and they are only seen at slaughter and post-mortem examination. Clinical signs supervene when the calculus obstructs the urethra and prevents the flow of urine. Castrated steers, having a very narrow urethra, are thus especially liable to this.

Obstructive urolithiasis is a fatal disorder. The affected animals commonly die of a ruptured bladder which bursts when it overfills. Uraemia follows and possibly also secondary infection. Round smooth stones are liable to cause complete obstruction of the urethra whilst irregular stones may inflict trauma on the bladder lining, which leads to cystitis and infection.

Acute pain is the predominant clinical sign. This is especially marked if the obstruction causes the retained urine to dam back and dilate the renal pelvis. The affected animal kicks repeatedly at its abdomen and makes repeated efforts to urinate, which results merely in the passage of a few drops of blood-stained urine. Precipitated crystals may be seen on the preputial hairs. Once the bladder ruptures the pain ceases, but is followed by uraemic depression, coma and death in a few days.

Diagnosis usually follows from appraisal of the clinical signs and frequently more than one animal may be involved in a group, making collective diagnosis easy. Prevention for the rest of the group is helped if the actual cause of the problem is identified, in particular the nutritional error which is involved. Analysis of the crystals in the urine generally indicates the chemical nature of the disorder. Blood chemistry may help to assess the phosphorus status.

Prevention and treatment

Obstructive urolithiasis needs surgical intervention. However, slaughter for salvage may be advisable if the animals are not uraemic or otherwise unsatisfactory for food. Medical treatment by change in diet is not generally successful and surgery of the bladder is not followed by a good prognosis.

Post-mortem examination of a slaughtered case may enable rational preventive measures for the surviving members of the herd. Most important, the calcium : phosphorus ratio must be balanced to prevent excess phosphorus excretion and precipitation in the urine. A Ca : P ratio of 2:1 has been recommended. Silicious calculi may be prevented by improving the water intake to increase the output of a more dilute urine. Adding salt to the ration has this effect (300 g daily for a 300 kg steer is said to be beneficial), by inducing diuresis.

The feeding of ammonium chloride (45 g/day) to steers has been found to prevent urolithiasis due to phosphatic calculi.

The danger of oxalate calculi can be circumvented by preventing access to oxalate-containing plants. Fortunately, female cattle do not seem to be prone to this type of calculus—presumably due to their wider urethra—and to a certain extent may consume this type of material with safety.

4/Disorders of water metabolism

Introduction

Metabolic disorders involving abnormal metabolism of water affect most of the major functions of the body. This is why the water content of the body's fluid compartments receives such careful control but once this regulation fails severe clinical signs and death rapidly supervene.

Water comprises about 70% of the body weight. All digestion and absorption in the alimentary tract takes place in a watery medium and all transport of metabolites occurs through the fluids of the blood and tissue spaces. Furthermore, waste materials are voided in urine with the aid of water excretion from the kidney. Water serves for cooling the body, especially in hot environments. It also maintains the mechanical rigidity of the soft tissues and organs.

In common with all metabolic disorders abnormality follows from imbalance between input and output, which in this case must lead to either dehydration or overhydration. Dehydration follows from deficiency of water intake, or from excessive loss in the faeces (as in diarrhoea), in urine (as in polyuria), or in sweat and panting to promote body cooling (as in high environmental temperatures). Abdominal disorders can also dehydrate because they interrupt the normal recycling of water from the digestive secretions.

In contrast, overhydration results from excessive drinking (possibly as an over-reaction to thirst), from kidney failure or as a terminal event in circulatory collapse when oedemal or ascitic fluid is not resorbed into the circulation.

Intake of water comes from several sources of which drinking is only one. Food itself contains water. Also, water derives from the catabolism of nutrients such as fats and carbohydrates (so-called metabolic water).

The output of water occurs via the faeces and urine, in respired air from the lungs and to a certain extent in cattle via sweat. Saliva tends to be overlooked as an output of water but several litres of saliva are secreted daily by cattle and should this fail to be resorbed lower down the intestines, as in various disorders and obstructions of the alimentary tract, then dehydration rapidly supervenes. Finally, output of water in the milk via the udder is an obvious necessity and vital if the lactating cow is to achieve productive output.

Water homeostasis depends on endocrinological control. Antidiuretic hormone (ADH) from the pituitary, secreted in response to increases in blood osmotic pressure, stimulates resorption of water from the kidney tubules. This system conserves water most effectively but leaves animals open to the danger of overhydration after thirst when they eventually obtain access to drinking water. Restoration of full regulatory function requires a few hours and during the interim too much water may be consumed. Other hormones involved include adrenal corticosteroids (which primarily affect sodium metabolism and water only secondarily) and sex hormones which cause cows to hydrate and dehydrate at various stages of the oestrous cycle.

Perhaps of greater importance than endocrinological factors is the thirst centre in the hypothalamus. This controls thirst and the actual intake of drinking water. A rise in blood osmotic pressure stimulates the desire to drink. This is especially important in cattle, which depend on sufficient water intake for the fermentation of food in the rumen by its flora and fauna. Not surprisingly, one of the first signs of water deprivation in cattle is a decline in appetite. Even so the rumen serves as a reservoir of water tiding the animals over temporary shortage whilst the hydration of the ruminal contents can be maintained by the flow of saliva.

Some cattle such as zebus survive for comparatively long periods without water. Several reasons account for this. These indigenous cattle develop behavioural patterns involving rest during the day, making maximal use of shade and grazing only at night or early morning when dew adds to the water intake. They are also adapted by being able to catabolize their body tissues and fat reserves to produce endogenous water, though at the expense of loss in weight and loss of production. Actually, the importance of endogenous water can be exaggerated because its production uses more oxygen which in turn means increased respiration and thus greater loss of water from the lungs. In hot environments endogenous water may only supply up to 20% of need and should not be overvalued as an important input.

Factors affecting water input

The nutritional need for water has been variously estimated. As a general rule cattle need free access to water to satisfy their thirst on demand. They then consume quantities which relate closely to their dry matter intake. Thus a restricted intake of water curtails appetite and vice versa. Although unrestricted access is the rule care is needed to ensure that this is a reality. Farmers commonly fail to realize that herds suffer deprivation of water without this being suspected. The reasons are many.

Dairy herds set up their own behavioural patterns for drinking, especially if they graze at a distance from the water troughs. They move up to drink collectively two or three times each day and if each tries to consume say 20 litres the trough soon empties and the inlet pipe may lack the capacity or head of pressure to replenish the supply fast enough. Although the leaders of the herd drink their fill, others may go thirsty until the next collective drink. The farmer who always sees a full trough may not realize that it empties too quickly for all the cows to drink their fill and some of them become dehydrated.

Cows differ from each other in their need for water. In fact, individual variation amounts to as much as 50% for no apparent reason. The quantity of dry matter eaten exerts an effect and so too does environmental temperature. For instance, at 40°C the water intake is 3.09 kg/kg food intake (as dry matter), at 60°C it is 3.84 kg/kg food intake, and at 80°C it is 5.17 kg/kg food intake. It is also important to note that European cattle (*Bos taurus*) drink more than Indian cattle (*Bos indicus*). Lactation imposes an additional burden, usually assessed at 50% extra need for water.

Calves automatically drink more than adults because of their predominantly liquid diets. Even so they need access to water to supplement their milk intake, especially if they are exposed to a warm environment. Also, milk replacer feeds may not always be mixed in the correct proportions and may be too concentrated. Diets for calves containing more than 15% dry matter result in reduced weight gain, particularly if there is even mild diarrhoea.

Certain diets affect the need for drinking water. Wet grass may contain over 80% water as compared with dry diets with only 5.7%. A high protein intake affects the need for water. Much of the protein converts to urea in the rumen and when excreted in the urine increases the need for water, possibly by over 25%. This occurs particularly in steers fed non-protein nitrogen supplements. Salt acts similarly, increasing water consumption by even 100%. This raises the important point that some water supplies contain salt; thus the cows must consume excess salt which has to be excreted via the urine. Some maintain that the salt content of drinking water should not exceed 1%. However, cows will tolerate even up to 1.3% without great harm. Over 2% leads to dehydration and lowered production.

Finally, the frequency of watering needs consideration. It is an important factor because cows with a continuous supply drink 18% more and yield more milk than those watered only once daily. Watering at increasing intervals has progressively deleterious effects. Compared with ad lib access, once daily watering reduces intake by 10% and once every other day by 31%. Uneven intakes are said to affect the concentration of the milk—massive intakes of water after milking, say in the morning, are said to cause a watery milk at the evening milking.

Farmers needing a 'rule of thumb' guide to water requirements usually assume a supply of 90 litres/cow/day as adequate. However, this figure may be misleading because the intake will be discontinuous as described above.

Factors affecting water output

Day-to-day control of water output depends on the regulation of urine excretion from the kidneys. However, with water deprivation the kidney tubules lack the power to concentrate urine above a maximum osmotic pressure. Urine, produced as a filtrate from the blood by the kidney glomeruli, is progressively concentrated in the tubules but only up to an osmotic pressure of 2.0 osmols. Although some species can concentrate even higher the cow cannot and thus some loss of water via the urine is obligatory.

Water output via the milk is an important factor in production. However, cows deprived of water reduce their milk output drastically to help maintain homeostasis. Quite modest deprivation reduces milk yield by 50% though the solids content of the secretion may be high. Thus the provision of a good water supply pays off from the point of view of economic production.

Faecal water is a major output because the cow produces copious quantities of very wet faeces of low osmotic pressure. This confers an advantage because in times of deprivation the cow can resorb water from its large intestine thus passing relatively dry faeces.

Water output can be high in hot weather to maintain cooling. Expired air is the major component but skin cooling is important in cattle because these animals possess a large number of sweat glands. In fact, the loss of water from the skin may be three times that from the lungs. Interestingly, indigenous cattle, adapted to hot environments, have more sweat glands than European breeds and thus presumably have an advantage.

The water compartments of the body

Total body water includes that circulating in the blood, that in the extracellular tissue spaces and that within the cells. This amounts to about 70% of body weight in cows and 85% in calves. Thin animals contain relatively more water than fat ones.

Various estimates suggest that an adult cow contains 4.2–4.8% of its body weight as blood. This implies that a 600 kg cow contains about 27 litres as blood volume. Blood consists of a mixture of cells and plasma. The cellular component is chiefly red blood cells which can be centrifuged into a layer to give a measure of hydration, known as the haematocrit. In cattle this normally varies between 23.4–34.4%. Values over 34.4% usually indicate progressively increasing degrees of dehydration. However, care must be taken over the interpretation of the test because water-deprived cows make every effort to conserve blood volume by reducing milk yield, resorbing water from faeces and withdrawing water from the tissue spaces until finally, when all other compensatory mechanisms are exhausted, the blood itself must undergo haemoconcentration and the haematocrit inevitably rises. Thus only in the later stages of dehydration is blood haematocrit an indicator of water deprivation.

Dehydration

Cattle become dehydrated in one of two ways. They may suffer deficient intake of water or excessive output. Deficient inputs commonly occur in hot arid regions but unfortunately they occur also in temperate areas with ample water supplies through failure of husbandry. Excessive output occurs principally in disorders such as diarrhoea.

Water deficiency

Cattle adapt well to temporary or mild water deprivation. Fluid intakes have to be intermittent in normal husbandry whilst output is to a large extent obligatory and continuous. Cattle meet this problem by using the water contained in the rumen and large intestine as reservoirs. However, relatively continued restriction seriously interferes with appetite and production and may soon give rise to clinical signs.

The cause

The precipitating cause of water deprivation is simply a shortage of supply. However, the implications of this need quantitative understanding. Restriction of intake by only 13% causes a nearly 10% reduction in milk yield, well before any clinical signs develop. A 60% restriction of normal water intake can still be compensated by decreases in urine volume and faecal water output. However, this is at the cost of secondary effects such as depressed appetite and reduction in milk yield. More severe deprivation of water (73–87% reduction of normal) causes severe inappetance with obvious clinical signs.

Rising temperature intensifies the effect of water deprivation. Increases in temperature provoke clinical signs with increasing rapidity. However, at 40°C animals can still compensate provided they have access to water. The animals drink 80% more water and increase sweating with the aid of increases in blood circulation and a lower haematocrit, which provides extra blood for circulation beneath the skin.

In hot arid countries the indigenous cattle avoid dehydration and need watering only once every 3 days—their water needs are said to be only half that of the Hereford breed. When severely deprived they can even withstand 2 months without water by fasting and metabolizing body fat. However, in these circumstances they merely survive and can hardly be described as productive.

Clinical signs and diagnosis

Thirsty cattle change in behaviour. They become excitable and knock down fences in frantic efforts to reach water. Undue excitability may be the first sign which leads the farmer to suspect water deprivation.

Physiologically, the initial response to dehydration is the withdrawal of fluid from the tissues to maintain blood volume. The faeces become dry and scanty. Appetite declines accompanied by drastic reduction in milk yield.

Progressive dehydration beyond the point of compensation inevitably leads to loss of blood volume and haemoconcentration with increased haematocrit. An early stage in the process can be detected by increased osmolarity of the blood and its electrolyte content. Later the blood becomes increasingly viscous and finally death occurs due to circulatory failure.

Other signs include loss of body weight—eventually up to 12%—with sunken eyes and loss of skin fold thickness and elasticity.

Diagnosis depends on detecting the behavioural changes and the typical clinical signs. The blood changes add confirmation; these include increased haematocrit and osmolarity. Also, blood urea rises because of the failure of the kidney to excrete the accumulating excess.

Prevention and treatment

Thirsty cattle drink copiously. Sudden access to water can lead to toxicity involving staggering, convulsions and even death. The problem is to exercise caution because cattle stampede in their wild endeavour to reach water. They drink large quantities very quickly; even moderate degrees of dehydration (say 10% loss of body weight) involve intakes of 40–50 litres of water for rehydration. Good husbandry is essential and it may be helpful to restrict drinking to small batches of stock when they are very thirsty.

It must be emphasized that cattle should have constant access to water both in the interests of their welfare, and also for them to achieve their potential for production.

Dehydration due to diarrhoea

Diarrhoea is a major cause of loss in calves. Although its principal aetiology consists of a large number and variety of infectious agents such as bacteria, viruses, cryptosporidia, etc., the actual cause of clinical signs and death follows from the loss of water in the diarrhoeic faeces. Provided the calves remain hydrated then most of them recover.

The cause

The dehydration accompanying diarrhoea resembles that due to water deprivation. Large quantities of body fluids drain into the diarrhoeic faeces. Compensation for this may be possible with the provision of ample drinking water, provided the sick calf maintains its water absorption. Homeostatic mechanisms give priority to maintaining blood volume. Thus the early stages of dehydration involve withdrawal of fluids from the tissue spaces and body cells. Eventually homeostasis fails and blood volume falls with increases in haematocrit, osmolarity and viscosity before the circulation breaks down and death supervenes. This classical type of dehydration is called hypertonic diarrhoea.

Other types of dehydration associated with diarrhoea occur which are either isotonic or hypotonic. This paradoxical situation is due to the following circumstances. In diarrhoea the calf loses not only water but also electrolytes and may lose weight because it breaks down its body tissues to supply its energy needs. There may be an overall deficit of water from the body—a true dehydration— but at the same time the blood may be relatively overhydrated. Factors such as transfer of extravascular water into the blood, destruction of red blood cells without their replacement, and a negative balance of protein coupled with hyperalbuminaemia all contribute to haemodilution and hypotonicity, even though the calf itself shows overall dehydration.

Normal calves have a total body water of about 87%, but this falls to 76% or even further in diarrhoea. Thus a calf weighing 40 kg needs 4 litres of water to re-establish its normal water content (see section on Treatment p. 53).

Clinical signs and death of calves from diarrhoea stem from several causes. First, circulatory collapse following increased blood viscosity is one possibility. Second, metabolic acidosis following kidney failure and unbalanced loss of electrolytes is another. Third, the breakdown of cells may allow potassium to leak into the circulation and the resulting hyperkalaemia induces cardiac arrhythmia and heart block. Cardiac fibrillation is a common terminal event. However complex the metabolic changes in diarrhoea the background problem is dehydration, which is why fluid replacement therapy is so vital a part of treatment.

Clinical signs and diagnosis

A calf with diarrhoea goes through a series of clinical stages all associated with its degree of dehydration. Only mild dehydration, involving merely 5% loss of body weight, shows some clinical signs such as sunken eyes and loss of skin elasticity. Even at this early stage the haematocrit may rise from the normal of 33% to 45%. At 7% loss of body weight the eyes are obviously sunken and the skin of the upper eyelid remains 'tented' when pinched into a skin fold. At 10% loss of body weight serious metabolic disturbances begin. The calf seems lifeless and unwilling to stand. It feels cold to the touch with a subnormal temperature. Beyond the stage of 10% loss of body weight circulatory efficiency falls and coma gradually supervenes with severe hypothermia, even as low as 29°C. The haematocrit varies. In hypertonic diarrhoea it may approach 55%, but many dying calves are hypotonic with low haematocrit values of even 25% or lower.

Diagnosis follows directly from the clinical signs. Blood chemistry may help in the choice of fluid therapy.

Prevention and treatment

Treatment depends on the stage of clinical signs. Merely mild dehydration indicates little need for fluid therapy, though antibiotics will be needed to combat infection. More severe dehydration requires fluid replacement on a relatively generous scale; as mentioned above a 10% loss of body weight is equivalent to 4 litres of replacement fluid. Five litres of a balanced electrolyte solution containing 5% dextrose given intravenously through a catheter over 24 hours has been found to give rapid recovery. However care is needed. Diarrhoeic calves lose sodium in their faeces, hence mere fluid therapy without sodium merely increases urinary excretion and deepens the hyponatraemia even further. An isotonic balanced electrolyte solution similar to the composition of normal plasma is recommended initially followed by a more appropriate formulation once the blood chemistry is known.

5 / Disorders of electrolyte metabolism

Introduction

The metabolism of sodium, potassium and chloride interrelates with several physiological systems in the body. First, these electrolytes control the osmolarity of the various compartments of water in the body and thus regulate the water contents of the tissue spaces and body cells. Second, sodium and potassium play a part in maintaining the electrical charge on cell surfaces and are vital for the ordered conduction of electrical impulses in nerves and muscles. Third, potassium has a vital role in certain enzymic interactions, especially those associated with energy metabolism. Fourth, both sodium and potassium help to control the acid–base status of the body. This is important not only for the control of acidity within the body proper but also for the regulation of fermentation within the rumen. The continuous flow of saliva, with its high content of sodium bicarbonate, neutralizes the acidity created by the ruminal flora and fauna as they digest the food intake.

Cattle are well adapted to sodium deficiency. They maintain sodium homeostasis for long periods on sodium-deficient diets without apparent harm. However, subclinical problems may ensue, especially related to digestive upsets and inefficient utilization of food intake. These can be just as important economically as the more overt clinical signs of pica which arise after long continued and severe sodium deficiency.

Metabolic upsets associated with derangement of sodium and potassium metabolism are typical examples of production disease. Indeed, modern intensive farming predisposes the cattle to imbalances in the input and output of electrolytes. Highly fertilized pasture usually contains far too much potassium for the needs of cattle, but these levels are necessary for optimum growth of grass which responds beneficially to much higher levels of potassium than those needed by grazing animals. In contrast, although herbage needs little sodium for good growth, lactating cows must have relatively large amounts. Modern grazing and cropping methods can predispose to the gradual removal and depletion of sodium from the pasture so that the cattle become more likely to suffer deficiency. This is made worse by the fact that milk contains an obligatory amount of sodium and should there be an outbreak of even mild subclinical mastitis the loss of sodium into the milk dramatically increases.

Modern husbandry may sometimes lead to excessive sodium intake. Intensively housed and fed animals have little or no control over their sodium intakes and may be forced to consume excess. Fortunately, this can be compensated if the animals have ample fresh water to allow any excess salt to be excreted in the urine. Examples of excess sodium intake occur when the animals graze salt marshes or receive dietary supplements of sodium bicarbonate to correct excess acidity in the rumen or in the silage.

Excess intake of potassium also occurs commonly. Although this may restrict magnesium absorption, in general it does little harm because the excess is excreted via the kidneys, explaining why urine from cattle is alkaline and contains large quantities of potassium bicarbonate.

Potassium deficiency rarely occurs in cattle, excesses of intake in herbage being the rule but the possibility does exist. In certain feedlot systems cattle may be fed on a high concentrate, cereal-based, diet with minimal roughage. Then potassium deficiency could occur.

Other ways in which deficiency of electrolytes may occur include diarrhoea, especially in newborn calves. This is important because many calves which now die could be saved if given properly balanced solutions of electrolytes.

Control of electrolyte homeostasis

Sodium is the most important cation circulating in the extracellular fluids such as the blood plasma, intercellular, or cerebrospinal fluids. In contrast, potassium is the predominant intracellular cation with a relatively low concentration in the extracellular fluids. The separation of the two electrolytes, sodium and potassium, across the cell wall is actively maintained and this determines the electrical potential on cell membranes of excitatory cells such as nerves and muscle fibres. Disruption of this balance creates acute problems of conductivity, thus precipitating paralysis and heart block.

Homeostasis of electrolyte metabolism varies in the closeness of its control, but sodium levels are so closely held that any minor departure from normal provokes instant and effective correction. The hormone aldosterone, released from the adrenal, corrects any tendency for hyponatraemia by conserving sodium from excretion. For instance, the loss of sodium via the urine or faeces can be virtually stopped. Also, potential losses of sodium in saliva can be circumvented by replacing sodium ions with potassium. So effective are these means for conserving sodium that clinical hyponatraemia supervenes only after prolonged periods of sodium deficiency when adjustments can go no further and homeostasis fails.

In contrast, potassium metabolism is not closely controlled. No clear hormonal mechanism for controlling concentrations in the blood seems to exist and any excess intake merely spills over via the kidney into the urine.

Table 5.1 contrasts the relative stabilities of sodium and potassium concentrations in the blood.

Plasma sodium concentration is far less variable than that of potassium. Even so seasonal hyponatraemia, though mild, is detectable in summer, presumably reflecting low sodium status on summer pasture as compared with that on indoor concentrate rations which are usually well supplemented with salt. As might be expected, day-to-day or diurnal variation of sodium concentration in blood is slight.

The total sodium content of a cow's body amounts to 1.39 g/kg or about 700 g in an adult animal. However, about 40–45% of this lies sequestered in bone where it binds onto the hydroxyapatite crystals. Here it seems to function as a reserve to be drawn upon in time of need. Another reserve of body sodium occurs in the

Table 5.1 Normal blood concentrations of sodium and potassium

	Normal mean concentration in blood plasma (meq/l)	Normal range (± 2SD)	Coefficient of variation (SD/mean)
Sodium	139	134–143	0.016
Potassium	5.0	4.3–5.7	0.070

rumen—indeed about half of the sodium ions in the extracellular fluid can be found in the rumen contents. Most of this flows in from the saliva. Cattle secrete vast quantities of saliva, up to 150 litres daily, containing 150 Eq/l of sodium as bicarbonate. This very large quantity represents five times the amount of sodium circulating in the entire blood plasma. Fortunately, virtually all this excreted sodium is efficiently resorbed back into the body either across the rumen wall or lower down the digestive tract. Thus virtually none is lost and the sodium contained in the recycling process can be considered as a temporary reserve giving a buffer to the loss of supplies in times of deficiency.

Sodium in the rumen has functions other than as a reserve. It maintains the osmotic pressure of the fluid within the rumen so that it stays at optimal pH for fermentation. In particular, it neutralizes the volatile fatty acids, acetic, propionic and butyric acids resulting from the fermentation of carbohydrates. This is why digestive function tends to fail in times of sodium deficiency.

Potassium, being primarily an intracellular cation, varies in total amount with the relative cellularity of the body. For instance, young and very muscular animals contain relatively more potassium than older fatter cows and the rapid growth of a young calf entails the need for a relatively large amount of potassium. The body content of adult cows is about 2.17 g/kg or a total of 1.09 kg. There are no reserves of potassium to be called upon in times of need as there are for sodium, but there is little need because cattle normally have the problem of coping with a relative excess and not with a shortage. For example, the daily needs of a dairy cow may be 30 g/day, but the actual intake may approach 500 g. When it is realized that an oral dose of 250 g of potassium as KCl can be fatal to a cow, it is surprising that potassium toxicity is not common.

Input/output relationships for electrolytes

Both sodium and potassium are fully absorbable from the alimentary tract. Sodium is actively absorbed against a concentration and electrochemical gradient. So effective is this that in time of sodium deficiency faecal sodium falls to nearly zero. In contrast, although potassium is also readily absorbed this is a passive process down a concentration or electrochemical gradient. Even so, potassium excretion in faeces is small (possibly only 0.3% of intake) the excess being almost entirely excreted in the urine.

Input/output relationships are dominated by the fact that most diets for cattle entail a relatively deficient sodium intake but a relatively excessive potassium intake. This is inevitable because the cow has evolved and is specialized to digest roughage intakes, the only problem being that with modern husbandry the sodium reserves of pasture become increasingly depleted whilst potassium levels are increasingly built up to secure maximum growth of herbage. Fortunately, as described above, cattle have evolved very good means for maintaining electrolyte homeostasis and can compensate for this inherent imbalance in their diets.

Extra problems arise when unusual outputs of electrolytes are superimposed on this well-balanced system. First, in young calves (and sometimes in adults too) diarrhoea imposes a massive drain on electrolyte reserves. Failure to resorb the sodium ions which are lost in the faeces can lead rapidly to sodium deficiency and dehydration due to the catastrophic fall in the osmotic pressure of extracellular water. Similarly, the loss of potassium in the exudates of the inflamed alimentary tract may even result in massive depletion of potassium and affected calves may die as a result of heart failure consequent upon hypokalaemia. In fact abdominal disorders of any kind, e.g. abomasal torsion or intestinal obstruction, may result in the accumulation of fluids and prevent the absorption of electrolytes lower down the alimentary tract.

Output of electrolytes in milk may also lead to metabolic problems for the dairy cow. Milk is a cellular secretion and thus has an intracellular type of ionic composition. In other words it is relatively rich in potassium, the concentration in milk even reaching 5–10 times that of blood plasma. Fortunately, the excessive intake of potassium mentioned above is more than sufficient to give cover for this. A far more difficult problem concerns sodium. Although concentrations of sodium in milk are usually low they are obligatory and can slowly deplete reserves in times of shortage. Furthermore, mastitis, even when only mild and subclinical, can create severe extra losses of sodium so that deficiency occurs even on apparently adequate intakes.

Problems of electrolyte deficiency

Sodium deficiency

A deficiency of sodium may occur from inadequate input, excess output, or a combination of the two. Small imbalances receive adequate correction under the influence of the adrenal hormone, aldosterone, but prolonged or severe deficiency eventually results in breakdown of homeostasis. Simple deficiency of sodium seldom gives rise to overt clinical signs under normal circumstances unless it is coupled with additional factors such as lactation, with or without mastitis, or in hot environments where losses of sodium in sweat become critical.

Cattle usually begin to show clinical signs after about 1 month of grazing on pasture containing less than 0.1 g sodium/100 g dry matter. Insidious signs at this stage include loss of appetite, usually for roughage before refusals of concentrates occur. Disappointing milk yields, ill-thrift and decreased body weight are also typical non-specific signs. Soon the general health deteriorates and the animals show anorexia, and look haggard with roughened coats.

A most dramatic clinical sign is pica. Sodium-deficient cattle strive to find salt. They lick each other, drink each other's urine and will even lick extensive excavations into soil in frantic efforts to find salt. In some herds this craving is accompanied by excessive drinking (polydipsia) and urination (polyuria). All cows in a herd may be involved in changed behaviour patterns, not only showing pica but also passing very pale urine every few minutes. It is assumed that loss of sodium leads to hypotonicity of the extra-cellular fluids which in turn affects the hypothalamus and decreases the secretion of antidiuretic hormone thus increasing the output of urine.

Other clinical signs occur. Undoubtedly sodium deficiency reduces milk yield very early on in the syndrome and it is also claimed that the fat content of milk is reduced. Furthermore, there may be an increased incidence of retained placentae and premature calvings. Correlations occur between sodium deficiency and infertility. However, these effects might be secondary and due to the reduced appetite and food intake.

Treatment and prevention of salt deficiency is simple. Theoretically the provision of at least 0.5% salt in the diet is considered adequate. However, for practical purposes allowing access to salt blocks is much more convenient. Two difficulties remain. Unrestricted access to salt either as a block or as a supplement mix can result in excessive intakes by individual animals and after a long period of deficiency a behavioural pattern resembling pica becomes established so that simple availability of salt may not always immediately reverse the clinical signs. Also the farmer must ensure adequate provision of fresh drinking water so that those animals which consume excess salt can excrete it in their urine to avoid salt poisoning.

Potassium deficiency

Naturally occurring deficiency of potassium is rare in cattle. Low potassium intakes, given experimentally, cause poor growth (probably due to potassium being a limiting factor for tissue and cellular development), reduced appetite, anaemia and diarrhoea. Eventually abnormalities in cardiac function supervene, probably related to degeneration in the Purkinje fibres of the myocardium.

Until recently there was a tendency to feed very large amounts of concentrates to dairy cows in order to increase production. These contained comparatively little potassium. As milk is a major route for the excretion of potassium the two factors might very occasionally combine and be enough to induce a genuine state of potassium deficiency. Certainly experimental diets containing only 0.06% K fed to dairy cows led to marked decrease in food intake, intense pica, loss of hair and skin condition and also fall in milk yield.

The diagnostic criterion for potassium deficiency is hypokalaemia. However, it must be stressed that potassium deficiency is not a practical problem and is practically unknown under conditions of normal husbandry and feeding.

Abdominal disorders as a cause of excessive output of electrolytes

In ruminants the most important causes of excess electrolyte loss are diarrhoea and certain kinds of intestinal obstruction. Newborn calves are especially liable to this because they suffer from diarrhoea due to certain toxigenic forms of *Escherichia coli* which allows fluid exudate in copious quantities to leak from the blood into the intestinal lumen from whence it passes out in the liquid faeces. Large quantities of sodium can be lost in this way and hyponatraemia becomes severe. This can be exacerbated if sodium-free dextrose solutions are used intravenously to replace the lost fluid volume because the sodium concentration and the osmolarity of the extracellular fluids will be decreased even further. This, when detected by the hypothalamus, results in the secretion of antidiuretic hormone, thus allowing loss of fluid via the kidneys so that the final outcome is severe dehydration, loss of blood volume and eventually circulatory collapse. This type of change is known as hypotonic dehydration. It is common in neonatal diarrhoea.

Diarrhoea gives rise to a complex sequence of events which involves loss of electrolytes other than sodium. For instance, loss of chloride and potassium occurs leading to hypochloraemia and hypokalaemia. Furthermore, the loss of chloride (and also of bicarbonate anions) can lead to a move in acid–base status towards acidosis. This complex of abnormalities can lead to complete breakdown in homeostasis and death unless prompt and adequate fluid replacement therapy is given. However, the clinician must decide what type of fluid therapy he should give for the maximum chance of recovery. For most purposes an isotonic solution containing a balanced mixture of electrolytes similar to that in normal plasma is recommended as a starting point. This can be given intravenously or orally depending on the clinical state of the case. The choice of other types of fluid appropriate to specific abnormalities such as acidosis depends on the assessment of blood chemistry to ensure that the chosen solution is not contraindicated. Good rates of cure are said to accompany fluid therapy in calves with diarrhoea, because most die of dehydration coupled with electrolyte depletion and imbalance. Fluid and electrolyte therapy should be designed to supplement antibiotic therapy in order to maintain homeostasis thus allowing the animal time to recover from the lesions of enteritis.

A similar complex sequence of changes occurs with obstruction of the alimentary tract. In these circumstances the metabolic derangement mainly involves chloride, which becomes trapped in the distended abomasum so that it cannot be recovered by absorption lower down in the intestines. This leads to electrolyte imbalance with hypochloraemia and alkalosis. Complications include hypokalaemia and dehydration. Surgical correction of the obstruction must of course be the primary objective, but a balanced electrolyte solution containing potassium and chloride (but with no bicarbonate) which is relatively acidic in reaction may speed recovery.

Excess input of electrolytes

Simple excess intake of sodium chloride can be toxic. In general, it is recommended that drinking water contains no more than 0.5% salt although 1% has been given without apparent harm. Signs of toxicity occur in cattle when the concentration in drinking water exceeds 1.75% though suboptimal weight gains occur when the concentration is as low as 1.25%. Even so, cattle will tolerate high intakes of salt provided they have access to ample supplies of fresh water.

The clinical signs of salt poisoning are mostly non-specific. Irritation of the intestinal mucosa provokes enteritis followed by diarrhoea. Also, the tissues of the body become dehydrated because of the accumulation of sodium chloride in the interstitial spaces. Chronic salt poisoning causes anorexia and polyuria, weakness and eventually collapse and death. In dairy cattle the anorexia may provoke ketosis—presumably because of the reduction in food input. Cerebral oedema occurs in some cases leading to convulsions before death supervenes.

Treatment simply consists of providing fresh water but care must be taken initially to avoid over-indulgence, which may temporarily exacerbate the physiological upset.

A special case of electrolyte imbalance occurs when sodium bicarbonate is used over-zealously to compensate for excess acidity in silage or to prevent ruminal acidosis on high concentrate diets. The problem is that the bicarbonate anion is metabolized leaving the sodium cation unbalanced and in relative excess. The problem need not give rise to overt clinical signs but the relative alkalosis induced in this way depresses bone metabolism and predisposes to milk fever. The reverse situation, notably feeding diets containing ammonium chloride, induces acidosis and increased bone metabolism; this has been used as a milk fever preventive.

6/Disorders of energy metabolism

Introduction

Energy metabolism is complex. Thus, not surprisingly, its associated metabolic disorders took a long time to unravel and only recently has a coherent account emerged. The problem is that the pathways of energy metabolism have a number of alternative routes and involve metabolites which can be used as replacement fuel in respiratory oxidation. Even so, glucose holds the central place. This is because it is vital for certain functions such as brain metabolism, the supply of lactose for milk production and the energy needs of metabolism in the liver.

The dominant position of glucose in energy metabolism presents difficulties for the ruminant because of this type of animal's peculiar biology. The presence of a rumen confers advantages in that poor-quality roughage feeds can be digested but this entails the disadvantage that almost no glucose is absorbed as the end-point of digestion. This is an important disadvantage as far as modern husbandry and heavily lactating cows are concerned.

In non-ruminants, carbohydrates such as starch are digested to glucose molecules as the sole end-products. These, after absorption, proceed directly to the liver and from thence to other body tissues for direct use as a respiratory fuel or for storage as fat or glycogen. In contrast, the ruminant is adapted to digest roughages and plant materials containing cellulose by fermentation in the rumen. Consequently, glucose is not an end-product of digestion and in fact the ruminant absorbs very little glucose from its alimentary tract. Fermentation by the micro-organisms in the rumen does not result in glucose but in volatile fatty acids such as acetic, propionic, and butyric acids. These are absorbed directly across the rumen wall for metabolism in the liver. Whilst it is true that propionic acid serves as a precursor of glucose, acetic and butyric acids do not, though they still find a place in energy production and can be stored as fat in adipose tissue.

Even for ruminants, glucose is an essential metabolite. They need steady inputs of glucose for their energy needs—just like non-ruminants—but must synthesize their own supplies from glucogenic precursors such as propionic acid, glucogenic amino acids from protein metabolism, and from glycerol which arises as a product of the hydrolysis of fats. Here lies the crucial problem. Can the high-yielding dairy cow, specially bred for milk production, make enough glucose for its needs? The special difficulty is that all the glucose required for the output of lactose in the udder must be made from glucose produced in the liver. If the liver fails to make enough then various metabolic disorders such as ketosis supervene.

Although ketosis is the major metabolic disorder of energy metabolism, other conditions include subclinical hypoglycaemia and the so-called 'fatty liver syndrome'. Both of these, like ketosis, are typical production diseases in the sense that they are induced by the combined strain of high production associated with inadequate or wrongly balanced feed input. The reverse type of disorder—that of excess input—needs mention at this stage. This is yet another production disease based on input/output imbalance but associated with over-rapid fermentation in the rumen which causes indigestion and metabolic acidosis.

Control of energy metabolism

Energy input

Carbohydrates consumed by cattle ferment to a mixture of volatile fatty acids (VFAs) under the enzymic activity of the ruminal microorganisms. On normal diets containing conventional roughage the proportions of VFAs produced are approximately 70% acetic, 20% propionic and 10% butyric acids. These proportions vary depending on the diet. A preponderance of starch or grain increases the proportion of propionic acid, and as this volatile fatty acid serves as a glucose precursor it enhances the animal's supply of glucose. Should abnormally large amounts of starch be eaten then the rumen reacts by producing large quantities of lactic acid. Although lactic acid is a normal though transient product of ruminal fermentation, excess of it, produced too rapidly, may temporarily exceed the capacity of the rumen to neutralize the acidity and a precipitate fall in pH results. Indigestion and metabolic acidosis are the consequence. However, lactic acid, just like propionic acid, is a glucose precursor and has the advantage that it can boost energy metabolism and glucose production in the liver.

Another problem arises when diets based on poor-quality roughage contain secondarily fermented silage. This may contain an excess of butyric acid which is not a glucose precursor and may even favour the development of ketosis because it is convertible into the ketone body, β-hydroxybutyrate.

Although cows do not normally absorb glucose directly from their alimentary tract, an exception occurs. Some types of carbohydrate, such as ground maize, partially escape ruminal fermentation and proceed into the small intestine for digestion to glucose under the influence of pancreatic amylase. The glucose so produced enters the body directly and boosts glucose supplies to give possible help in any impending problem of ketosis.

Volatile fatty acids form the major source of energy input for cattle. Acetic acid, though predominant, does not yield glucose in the body's metabolic pathways. However, it is used as a respiratory fuel by a variety of tissue cells, but only if adequate supplies of glucose are available from alternative sources. Acetic acid can also be built up into triglycerides and be stored as fat in the body's reserves or it can be used for the production of milk fat in the udder, again provided glucose is available for the synthesis of the glycerol part of the lipid molecule.

Propionic acid must be viewed as the most important precursor of glucose absorbed as a product of ruminant digestion. It probably contributes as much as 30–50% of the total glucose supply, the bulk of the remainder coming from glucogenic amino acids (25%) and lactate (15%). Thus propionic acid has the major part to play in maintaining the pathways of energy metabolism in the cow.

In contrast, butyrate contributes no glucose. It rapidly crosses the rumen wall where most is converted to the ketone body β-hydroxybutyric acid which, theoretically at least, adds to ketosis susceptibility. However, ketones are not necessarily dangerous metabolites. In normal circumstances they can be used as a respiratory fuel in tissues such as cardiac and skeletal muscles. Indeed ketones provide a normal source of energy in cows. The difficulty comes in time of temporary food deprivation when the body has to mobilize its reserves. This gives rise to very little glucose compared with the needs of lactation. Then alternative pathways for energy supply come into play which involve the production of ketones, which cannot be used unless there is adequate glucose. Initially, the deprived cow enters a phase of controlled ketogenesis which can continue satisfactorily until the whole metabolic system fails when supplies of glucose run out.

Various factors adversely affect the input and use of volatile fatty acids. First, deficiency of vitamin B_{12} interferes with carbohydrate metabolism by inhibiting the conversion of propionic acid into glucose in the liver. Another factor concerns the activity and function of the ruminal flora and fauna. Any circumstance that upsets homeostasis within the ruminal contents adversely affects the fermentation processes. For instance acidity needs control. Hence, continuous flow of saliva is vital because, should its buffering function fail, immediate indigestion and metabolic acidosis results. Also the normal osmolarity of the rumen contents needs control. Hence adequate intake of electrolytes, especially that of sodium, needs priority. Finally, the ruminal flora and fauna need adequate nutritional supplies. Without this they cannot thrive and carry out their normal digestive function. This means that sufficient protein and appropriate trace elements must be available for their multiplication and activity. See Fig. 6.1 for a schematic drawing of energy input in rumen fermentation.

Energy output

The special needs of the pregnant cow and the lactating udder impose obligatory demands on glucose supplies. Lactose is made almost exclusively from glucose molecules and up to 2 kg must be synthesized daily in the liver. In addition, glucose forms a vital component in the synthesis of glycerol for milk fat. Between 70–90% of a cow's total supply of glucose is needed by lactation alone, leaving little left over for the other obligatory needs for glucose in brain metabolism, synthesis of body fats and respiratory oxidation in the tricarboxylic acid cycle, which is vital for energy provision in all body cells.

Control of energy metabolism

The central factor in preventing disorders of energy metabolism is the regulation of homeostasis in the supply and demand for glucose. Normally this receives effective control by hormones. If the cow becomes hyperglycaemic then insulin secreted by the pancreas reduces blood glucose by inhibiting glucose synthesis

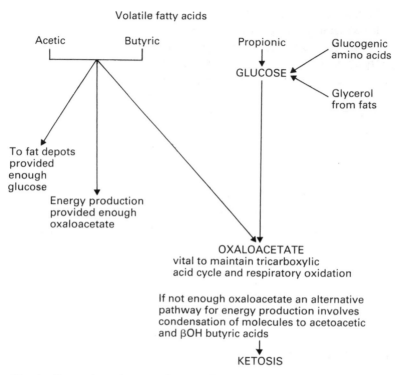

Fig. 6.1 Energy input in rumen fermentation.

(gluconeogenesis) in the liver and also by stimulating the uptake and storage of glucose within cells either as glycogen or fat. In cattle, insulin secretion occurs not only as a result of hyper-glycaemia, but also by rises in blood VFA concentration—hardly surprising as VFAs form such an important part of the ruminant input of energy.

Conversely, hypoglycaemia induces the secretion of glucagon coupled with a decrease in insulin. In addition, glucoreceptors in the hypothalamus also respond and stimulate epinephrine secretion from the adrenal. The combined effect of this hormonal response to hypoglycaemia is to release glucose from glycogen stores in the liver, mobilize glycerol and free fatty acids from fat reserves, and mobilize amino acids from protein reserves in muscles.

The hormones glucagon and epinephrine work rapidly. Longer-term responses are controlled by other hormones, including growth hormone and adrenocorticotrophic hormone (ACTH), secreted from the pituitary gland, which releases glucocorticoids from the adrenal cortex. Growth hormone initially works like insulin by favouring glucose mobilization and fat storage, but in the longer term it increases mobilization from fat stores and stimulates milk production. Glucocorticoids on the other hand stimulate gluconeogenesis in the liver and thus enhance the supply of glucose for the lactating mammary gland.

An important control factor for the homeostasis of glucose in the lactating cow is that hypoglycaemia results in decreased production of milk. Clearly, this self-correcting response spares the output of glucose in time of temporary shortage, but not entirely in the interests of the farmer who depends on profitable milk production. The other problem is that this fail-safe mechanism can be over-ridden. In early lactation the hormones stimulating milk secretion take predominance and the cow continues to secrete copious quantities of milk even though she is hypoglycaemic.

Ketosis

Introduction

Ketosis is a typical example of production disease. It results from an input/output imbalance in energy metabolism. Consequently, it is liable to occur when lactation and energy requirements reach a peak. The disease is variously called acetonaemia, slow fever, postparturient dyspepsia, hypoglycaemic ketosis, etc. These names characterize different aspects of the syndrome but basically ketosis of dairy cows is a metabolic disorder occurring in early lactation and associated with hypoglycaemia, ketonaemia, ketonuria, inappetence, loss of weight and incoordination. Some animals show neural signs of either lethargy or even excitability.

It is a relatively common condition. Some 10% of the cows in early lactation may be ketotic in certain herds with many animals showing various degrees of severity in clinical signs. Fortunately, very few die because in due course the disease self-corrects, milk yield falling with eventual spontaneous recovery. However, the economic losses due to the interference with production remain.

The cause

It is generally agreed that ketosis is an extreme degree of the normal state of high-yielding dairy cows. All of them suffer negative energy balance in early lactation and most adapt satisfactorily to this situation, but for some a comparatively mild adverse event converts subclinical hypoglycaemia into a genuine case of ketosis with clinical signs. Most cows just cannot eat enough food for their energy needs in lactation and depend on mobilizing their fat reserves to make good the deficiency with consequent risk of ketosis.

The central determining factor is blood glucose concentration. Hypoglycaemia is the factor which eventually triggers ketosis. The sequence of events appears to be as follows:

1 The need for lactose in the lactating mammary gland initiates a shortage of glucose which in turn limits the production of a key metabolite in the tricarboxylic acid cycle, oxaloacetate.

2 Shortage of oxaloacetate inhibits the use of the tricarboxylic acid cycle for energy production.

3 To maintain energy output the cow uses an alternative, but potentially inefficient, metabolic pathway leading to acetoacetic and β-hydroxybutyric acid production.

4 Mobilization of reserves from adipose tissue leads to liver cells accumulating excess droplets of fat which fail to be metabolized, presumably because of shortage of glucose and other metabolites needed for fat transport. Eventually the liver becomes overloaded with fat and undergoes fatty degeneration with decline in function and an even lower capacity to synthesize glucose.

5 The energy metabolism of the cow now starts an irreversible decline, or vicious circle, from which relief can only come from new supplies of glucose, or a fall in glucose output by a dramatic decrease in the demands of milk production.

A key factor in this hypothesis is that oxaloacetate is a vital link in the supply of energy by the tricarboxylic acid cycle. This cycle is essential not only for respiratory oxidation, but also for glucose synthesis. Thus, should this cycle fail, the animal is progressively deprived of its capacity to generate fresh supplies of glucose for milk production. It is then forced to use the alternative ketogenic pathways to satisfy its energy needs.

In the simplest terms, ketosis results from the difficulty of the high-yielding cow in providing glucose for milk lactose coupled with the fact that glucose is vital for the synthesis of replacement supplies in the liver and, also, to keep the tricarboxylic acid cycle fully active.

Not every high-yielding cow suffers from ketosis. Hence, some factors must operate which increase susceptibility. First, the disorder seems to be associated with intensive farming, especially when cows are housed during the winter and may lack exercise. It is also especially common in cows that become over-fat in late pregnancy. Second, certain types of silage seem to be involved, especially those containing large quantities of butyric acid. Third, factors affecting appetite may be superimposed. In some herds a deficiency of cobalt or phosphorus seems to be important. Fourth, certain breeds and certain individuals within breeds are especially susceptible, indicating a possible genetic link. Finally, secondary ketosis commonly results from any reduction in dietary intake consequent upon an abdominal disorder, metritis or mastitis.

Clinical signs and diagnosis

The earliest clinical sign is some reduction in milk yield and a smell of acetone in the cow's breath, milk and urine. At this stage no other overt signs may appear and the cow recovers spontaneously. However, if severity progresses the appetite fails, though initially this may involve only refusal of concentrates whilst normal intake of silage and hay continues. Soon a critical point is reached. Body weight rapidly falls, mainly due to loss of body water, the faeces become dry and hard, and the cow begins to look miserable and depressed. Other clinical signs include decreased ruminal movements. Sometimes nervous signs appear, often suddenly. The cow may walk in circles and even seem to be blind. On occasion the signs may progress to resemble milk fever with paresis and collapse.

Diagnosis depends finally on blood chemistry. Hypoglycaemia is always present coupled with ketonaemia (usually measured as β-hydroxybutyric acid). A common screening test involves pouring a little freshly-drawn milk onto Rothera powder and observing a simple colour reaction for a positive result. Large numbers of milk samples can be monitored in the dairy parlour by this test and any early case set aside for treatment before clinical signs have time to supervene. In some herds over 10% of recently calved cows may react positively and require treatment to maintain milk yield if not clinical health.

Prevention and treatment

Prevention depends on avoiding any condition predisposing to failure of intermediary metabolism. A ten point plan exists for general use:

1 Avoid over-fatness in late lactation.
2 Prevent over-fatness in the dry period.
3 'Steaming up' should be limited to only 4–5 weeks before calving.
4 Gradually increase food intake for lactation.
5 Increase the concentrates gradually in line with milk yield.
6 Use a balanced concentrate ration containing not more than 16–18% protein. The addition of some ground maize has special advantages because some escapes rumen fermentation. It can be digested and absorbed directly as glucose.
7 Avoid interrupting normal routines and access to food—allow enough time for all of the ration to be eaten.
8 Keep the constituents of the ration constant.
9 After peak lactation the highly digestible carbohydrates can be gradually replaced with cheaper cereals.
10 Ensure the palatability of the roughage. Avoid badly made silage.

Finally, it is recommended that the high-yielding cows be monitored regularly for ketones in the milk by the Rothera test so that treatment can be speedily put in hand.

Treatment commonly involves the use of glucocorticoids or ACTH. ACTH stimulates the adrenal to produce its own glucocorticoid so that both treatments act similarly, by stimulating the tricarboxylic acid cycle and also gluconeogenesis from glucogenic amino acids. Anabolic steroids are also highly effective.

Intravenous glucose solutions give a direct supply of glucose but this beneficial effect is merely transient. Intravenous drips have advantage for a more continuous supply but are cumbersome under practical conditions. Oral treatments with sodium propionate and propylene glycol can be efficacious—both are rapidly absorbed and converted to glucose in the liver. So too is molasses given orally as a drench.

Should a nutritional deficiency be probable then this needs correction; vitamin B_{12} or cobalt being the most likely suspects.

Fatty liver syndrome

Introduction

This condition appears to be increasing in prevalence. Surveys using liver function tests suggest that 30–40% of cows may suffer fatty liver of sufficient severity to be termed pathological. Although such cows may show no overt clinical signs they tend to be infertile with delayed onset of ovarian cycles after parturition.

The cause

The cause of fatty liver shares many similar features with those of ketosis. Both involve a negative energy balance in early lactation. However, fatty liver is really due to the excessive mobilization of fat from the adipose tissue and thus fat cows appear to be especially susceptible. Much of the problem stems from excess feeding in late pregnancy so that the fat depots become over-replete. The condition is not confined to lactating cows, but can occur in beef animals also, in particular in cows carrying twin calves and thus tending to negative balance in energy. Much of this is caused by over-fatness brought on when grazing good summer pastures which become depleted in nutritional value in autumn. Although relatively few cows are affected clinically by the condition mortality can be high, up to 10% or more in certain herds.

The pathogenesis of the fatty liver is as follows. There is excessive mobilization of fat, mainly in the form of free fatty acids from the fat depots. This increases the concentration of fatty acids in the blood which, on transport to the liver, condense into fat droplets in the liver cells. The liver cells become so grossly distended with fat that their metabolism is slowed and they undergo degeneration. Finally, liver function fails and the cow may die.

Clinical signs and diagnosis

The disorder occurs typically in fat cows shortly after they calve. Usually a precipitating factor can be identified such as indigestion or some other abdominal disorder. The cow may totally fail to eat and develop severe ketosis with death in a few days. Some cows survive and recover but remain infertile for long periods.

Blood chemistry shows a variable series of abnormalities. First and foremost, liver enzymes leak from the damaged cells and can be found in the blood, the concentration depending on the severity of the liver damage. Diagnostically these enzymes include glutamic oxaloacetic transaminase (GOT), ornithine carboxyl transferase (OCT) and sorbitol dehydrogenase (SDH). Second, ketonaemia is usual and also varying degrees of hypocalcaemia. Mild, but chronic, cases show hypoalbuminaemia indicating a long-term failure of liver function.

If death occurs a necropsy reveals the severity of fatty change in the liver which is grossly enlarged, yellow and greasy with fat. The kidney tubules and heart wall will probably also be loaded with fat droplets.

Prevention and treatment

The principal aim is to prevent pregnant cows from becoming over-fat. This is not always easy to achieve because on pasture, or even indoors, some cows tend to be greedy and eat more than others. Combating this means dividing cows into small groups based on condition and then feeding according to need. Metabolic profiles detect animals on the verge of a clinical disorder needing special treatment. Every effort must be made to maintain appetite and energy intake after calving.

Effective treatment needs prompt application. Parenteral glucose and calcium borogluconate assist recovery especially for cows which still continue to eat. Glucocorticoids and vitamin B_{12} are commonly used, but their value depends on the severity of liver pathology. Recovery or maintenance of appetite usually signals a successful outcome.

It must be stressed that many cows undergo a period of mild fatty change in the liver after calving. Although most show no clinical signs it must be assumed that such animals are finely balanced on a 'knife edge'—the superimposition of a factor reducing food intake could precipitate a fatal outcome. In any case treatment of fatty liver remains wise because of the relationship to infertility.

Metabolic acidosis

Introduction

Metabolic acidosis in cattle commonly follows excess intake of highly fermentable carbohydrates. These can ferment in the rumen to yield lactic acid at such a rate that the normal processes of acid neutralization are overwhelmed. This leads to various metabolic problems but, in particular, the metabolic health of cattle depends on the maintenance of proper levels of fermentation by the ruminal micro-organisms. Sudden changes in acidity of the rumen contents give rise to inappetance and indigestion as well as to systemic acidosis.

As already discussed, carbohydrates ferment in the rumen to a mixture of the volatile fatty acids, acetic, propionic and butyric. Lactic acid is also produced, but usually in only small transitory amounts. However, should the ruminant eat too much readily fermentable material the growth of lactic acid-producing bacteria is enhanced so that they dominate the normal flora and fauna of the rumen. The excess lactic acid may sometimes accumulate to such an extent that it corrodes the rumen wall, inflicting large areas of necrosis on its epithelial lining. Furthermore, on absorption from the rumen, the lactic acid induces systemic metabolic acidosis.

Metabolic acidosis may be acute or chronic. Acute forms of the disorder occur by the accidental ingestion of excessive quantities of starch or grain. A group of stock may break out of confinement. If they enter a food store they may gorge themselves on a wide range of carbohydrate foodstuffs. Underfed animals are particularly susceptible. Some overeat even when fed normal quantities because dominant cattle eat selfishly and consume more than their share. They may suffer acute indigestion while the rest of the stock remains normal.

In contrast, chronic indigestion occurs in fattening stock fed unbalanced diets containing minimal (or unpalatable) roughage coupled with highly concentrated feed. The barley beef system of fattening illustrates a typical situation. The continued intake of large quantities of barley leads to undesirable fermentation in the rumen which induces chronic acidosis and unthriftiness. Although this system is now rarely used, animals may still be aggregated into large feedlots where unlimited access to concentrate feed allows the greediest of them to eat excessively.

The cause

The cause of acute metabolic acidosis is almost always carbohydrate engorgement. The toxic effect of this depends on the rapidity of fermentation; thus finely ground material tends to be more dangerous than whole grains. The immediate cause is accumulation of excess lactic acid in the rumen. In normal circumstances the concentration of this metabolite in the rumen is low. The same is true of lactic acid in the blood, which is kept low because it is avidly taken up by liver cells. Lactate is also used by several other cells in the body. It is a source of energy and a precursor of glucose. Normally the rate of utilization more than copes with the rate of lactate input. If it does not, then lactaemia and acidosis develop as a metabolic disorder.

The normal rate of lactic acid input into the rumen amounts to about 750 g/day from conventional roughages such as silage but the normal flow of saliva with its phosphate buffer easily copes with its neutralization. Lactic acid produced by the rapid fermentation of grain can overload this mechanism. Toxic doses of carbohydrate are variously estimated. For instance, dairy cows which are accustomed to concentrate rations can consume 15–20 kg of grain with little harm but beef cows on pasture, unaccustomed to grain diets, may die after eating only 10 kg of grain. It seems that the microorganisms of the rumen adapt only relatively slowly to dietary intake and are susceptible to sudden change. Even normal intakes can be toxic if the animals gorge after missing one of their daily feeds and then make up for it by consuming the full daily ration all at once.

The sequence of events appears to be as follows:

1 Within a few hours of eating highly fermentable food the population of micro-organisms in the rumen changes. *Streptococcus bovis* assumes predominance and produces large quantities of lactic acid and will continue to do so even though the rumen pH falls to 5 or even less. At this pH the other bacteria and protozoa are killed but the low pH allows lactobacilli to multiply and produce even more lactic acid.

2 The excess lactic acid increases the osmolarity of the ruminal contents so that water leaves the blood and causes dehydration.

3 The animal attempts to buffer the ruminal acidity with saliva and by the removal of bicarbonate from the blood plasma. This reduces

the alkaline reserve. Lactic acid is also absorbed directly into the blood thus reducing the alkaline reserve still further and causing metabolic acidosis.

4 Ruminal fermentation produces both D- and L-forms of lactic acid. The L-lactic acid causes less harm because it is rapidly metabolized leaving the D-isomer to accumulate. Thus the D-form of lactic acid is the more dangerous because the animal metabolizes it only very slowly.

5 Lactic acid is corrosive to the ruminal wall, large segments of which may die and be sloughed. This allows fungal and bacterial infection to invade and set up ruminitis. In severe cases gangrene may supervene and infection may even penetrate to cause peritonitis.

6 Even mild lactic acid poisoning causes stasis of the rumen and allows infection to enter through the damaged rumen wall with liver abscesses as the result. Chronic acidosis in the rumen causes considerable lesions of hyperkeratosis of the wall and liver degeneration.

7 It has been stated that some toxins such as histamine or bacterial endotoxin contribute to the toxic effect of ruminal acidosis. The role of these remains uncertain.

Clinical signs and diagnosis

The severity of signs depends on the circumstances of the engorgement. Sudden introduction of rapidly fermentable carbohydrate to susceptible cattle is quickly fatal. On the other hand, a gradual onset of chronic signs follows toxicity from planned diets containing a moderate excess of cereals.

The first clinical signs after acute engorgement consist of enlarged rumen size and abdominal spasms of pain coupled with reluctance to eat. Ruminal movements slow down and the animals cease to ruminate.

Within 24 hours the affected animals may stagger and soon collapse. Some appear drunk or partially blind. The heart rate is generally high, especially so in animals that will probably die. Failure to defaecate is thought to be another grave sign but many animals suffer a profuse diarrhoea.

Dehydration progressively supervenes and in cases where the kidney tubules degenerate there may be anuria.

Blood chemistry can give helpful information for prognosis and treatment. Haemoconcentration gauges the extent of dehydration —the haematocrit may rise to 50% in severe cases. Blood lactate levels may be measured to confirm the acidosis and predictably the blood pH and bicarbonate levels will be low. The pH of ruminal fluid gives guidance—less than pH 5 indicates a severe case unless the animal is accustomed to a cereal diet and a low rumen pH.

Severe cases die in 1–2 days. Survivors may succumb later to the secondary effects of ruminitis and infection. Recovered animals may show chronic laminitis, the cause of which is not entirely clear, but could be due to vascular constriction of the blood supply to the hoof corium.

Prevention and treatment

Prevention depends on avoiding circumstances where engorgement can occur. However, fattening stock may be fed on cereal-based diets quite satisfactorily provided they are given time to adapt gradually. The roughage content of the ration must be maintained in the early stage of adaptation, preferably in a roughage/cereal mixture to prevent engorgement. This inhibits greedy animals eating far more of the cereal than their calculated share.

Buffers can be added to the diet. Sodium bicarbonate is commonly used for this purpose especially during the stage of adaptation. It is said to prevent mild subclinical effects which interfere insidiously with growth rate. Antibiotics have also been used to suppress lactic acid-producing bacteria in the rumen.

Finally, successful prevention of acidosis is said to follow the 'inoculation' of unadapted cattle with ruminal fluid from those that have been on cereal diets for some time. This fluid contains bacteria capable of the rapid uptake and metabolism of excess lactic acid in the rumen.

Treatment depends on correcting the ruminal and systemic acidosis. In its early stages this means removing the animals from access to the feed which has caused the problem. Good quality hay should be offered and mild exercise may help stimulate the onward movement of the ingesta.

Animals showing severe clinical signs with anorexia, depression and dehydration need special treatment. Free access to water can lead to fatal consequences—the cows may drink excessively and die from electrolyte imbalance. Rumenotomy is the most radical procedure but likely to be successful. The contents of the rumen are removed and the rumen washed out with water. The rumen then needs reseeding with cud from a healthy cow to restore normal fermentation.

Systemic metabolic acidosis can be treated with intravenous infusions of isotonic (1.3%) sodium bicarbonate. The same solution can be used directly via a cannula into the rumen, though other alkalizing agents such as magnesium oxide may be preferable and more immediately effective by this route. In some cases, affected by paresis and hypocalcaemia, intravenous calcium borogluconate may help speed recovery. Other possible therapies include antihistaminics (for laminitis) and gut stimulants to encourage alimentary activity and maintain appetite.

7/Nitrogen or protein metabolism

Introduction

Ruminants are favoured nutritionally because, with a rumen, they can synthesize protein from non-protein sources of nitrogen. The ruminal micro-organisms perform this function by degrading the nitrogenous components of the food into ammonia which they then build up into bacterial protein and eventually, when the ruminal protozoa ingest bacteria, into protozoal protein. This newly-formed protein passes into the abomasum and intestines for digestion and absorption in the form of amino acids, just as in non-ruminant digestion. The advantage for the ruminant is that it does not depend on high-quality protein and can use the poor-quality material in roughage. There is yet another advantage. Any urea, formed as a waste product of protein metabolism within the animal's body, can be recycled via the saliva for reuse as a protein source in the rumen. This recycling process enables cattle to economize on protein intake. In addition, from the practical point of view, cheap non-protein nitrogen compounds such as urea can be used to supplement the ruminant's dietary intake. Theoretically at least, cattle thrive on diets containing almost no actual protein at all, but unfortunately there are metabolic problems which then ensue.

Three main problems can be identified. First, the ruminal micro-organisms need at least some protein for their own well-being, multiplication and activity. They fail to thrive on completely non-protein intakes. Second, the nitrogen recycling processes via the saliva and the rumen are not very efficient. Some ammonia and urea is inevitably lost by excretion in the urine and the protein in bacterial cells in the rumen (especially that associated with nucleic acids) resists digestion. There are even some advantages in by-passing degradation of protein in the rumen, especially for high-yielding dairy cows which depend on generous intakes of concentrates for production. Indeed, diets containing a proportion of undegradable protein confer special value for high-yielding dairy cows. Third, the activities of the ruminal micro-organisms impose a penalty. Should the cows gain access to excessive quantities of rapidly degradable protein or urea they can suffer from ammonia poisoning.

Control of protein metabolism

Input/output factors

In general, 50–80% of proteinaceous material in cattle fodder is degraded in the rumen to ammonia and then converted into microbial protein. The degradable percentage in silage exceeds that in most feeds. Proteins such as zein in maize which are relatively undegradable pass almost unchanged into the abomasum for enzymic digestion lower in the alimentary tract.

Although ammonia is a potential toxic hazard it is only so if present in harmful excess. Concentrations are usually kept low because as rapidly as ammonia is produced it is avidly removed by bacteria for rebuilding into protein. The speed at which this removal occurs depends on the energy provided to the bacteria by the fermentation of carbohydrates, which also supply the vital carbon skeletons for the synthesis of amino acids within the bacteria. Thus protein and energy metabolism are closely intertwined in the ruminant. A deficiency of the one leads to deficient utilization of the other.

This complex balanced system for the input of proteinaceous compounds works smoothly provided there is a steady input of forage. It becomes disordered when the composition of the feed suddenly changes.

When ammonia is produced by the degradation of protein in the rumen most of it is normally taken up by the ruminal bacteria. However, some passes directly through the rumen wall and thus to the liver via the portal blood vessels where it is converted into urea. In normal circumstances the liver removes ammonia most efficiently because the ammonia concentration in the peripheral circulation is kept very low. In contrast, blood urea varies depending on protein intake. It appears to have no ill effects and many investigators find that its concentration in the blood gives a useful measure of protein status—a cow on low protein intakes may have a blood urea as low as 2 mg/100 ml rising to 30 mg/100 ml on high intakes of protein. There appears to be no effective homeostatic control.

Blood urea cannot be used within the body as a source of protein but it occupies a central place in the nitrogen economy of the animal. Its fate depends on the animal's protein status. In time of excess protein intake blood levels of urea rise and increasingly large amounts spill over into the urine. Recycling of blood urea back into the rumen also depends on blood concentrations. Urea enters the ruminal fluid across the rumen wall down a concentration gradient and thus more recirculates at higher concentrations of blood urea. The same is true for urea in the saliva.

The building blocks of proteins are the amino acids. These are the end-products of protein digestion in the abomasum and the small intestines. The liver can synthesize some of them and hence these are called non-essential amino acids. Some the liver cannot make and these are essential in the sense that they have to be absorbed from the intestines in their final form. The rumen bacteria can synthesize all of the essential amino acids, though the proportions are not necessarily optimal for high production of milk. The amino acid composition of rumen bacteria stays reasonably constant and thus the rumen tends to modify the ingested protein to a relatively standard type. An important exception to this rule is that protozoa tend to produce protein of a higher digestibility and quality with a higher component of the essential amino acid, lysine; hence, diets favouring protozoal proliferation improve the proportions of amino acids available on digestion.

Individual amino acids serve separate functions. For instance, glycine (amounting to 20% of total intake of amino acids) is used for glucose synthesis and also for the detoxification of benzoic acid. Glutamate finds importance in the detoxification of ammonia. Alanine is a precursor of glucose. Indeed, up to a third of glucose needed for high milk yields may derive from glucogenic amino acids. On the other hand, methionine plays an important and possibly rate limiting part in the synthesis of milk casein. It is also a methyl group donor in the synthesis of lipoproteins and hence may thus help in the prevention of fatty liver and ketosis.

The concentration of amino acids in blood is very low (only about 50–60 μg/ml) but throughput is extremely rapid so that continuity of supply must be secured. Theoretically, the concentration of individual amino acids in the blood could indicate metabolic status, but in practice this is rendered impossible because concentration gives little indication of availability with such an active throughput. Many amino acids have a half life in the blood of only a few minutes.

Tissue, and especially muscle, proteins form an important and labile source of amino acids. This is important because lactation imposes such a severe demand on protein resources that it can seldom be met by dietary intake alone, with the result that catabolism of muscle protein becomes inevitable. But it must be replenished in the dry period. Cows can lose considerable amounts of muscle in early lactation. Hopefully this builds back when the period of negative balance ends. However, muscle cells, in contrast to fat cells in the fat depots, possess limited powers of replication and regeneration, especially in adult life. How far can cows maintain an adequate muscle mass after repeated lactations? The answer is unknown.

Other components of the body involved in the metabolism of protein include the blood proteins, haemoglobin, albumin and globulin. Of these, albumin is synthesized in the liver from amino acids. Thus, hypoalbuminaemia results not only from protein deficiency with inadequate supply of amino acids, but also from malfunction of the liver with degeneration or fatty change. Both situations commonly occur at the same time during early lactation. Fortunately, serum albumin is catabolized slowly and only gradually falls in concentration as it fails to be replaced. A period of at least one month is needed before significant change takes place.

Haemoglobin reacts similarly. It is synthesized in the blood cell-forming tissues of the bone marrow, but in time of protein deficiency this activity declines so that the concentration of blood haemoglobin falls resulting in anaemia. Other interacting factors in malnutrition, which also cause anaemia, include trace elements such as iron, copper and cobalt, all three being needed for haemoglobin synthesis.

Globulins confer immunological competence. High concentrations in blood (hyperglobulinaemia) commonly link with recent immunological events such as infectious disease or vaccination. Hypoglobulinaemia on the other hand, usually indicating low immunological competence, occurs in calves which do not receive sufficient supplies of globulin from the colostrum.

Albumin, and to some extent globulin, need effective homeostatic control because they influence the osmolarity of blood. Thus the concentration of the two go hand in hand, e.g. hypoglobulinaemia may be compensated by a corresponding increase in blood albumin and vice versa. This compensating effect may not be complete because albumin has roughly twice the osmolarity of globulin.

The loss of proteins from the body follows various routes. The most important is that from the udder which must synthesize milk casein. Milk contains about 3.5% protein so that the total daily output amounts to over 1 kg in a cow giving 30 kg of milk daily. This highlights the burden of heavy lactation because one day's output of milk roughly equates with the 1 kg of albumin circulating in the blood of the cow. It is not surprising that lactation commonly requires 15 kg of protein to be removed from the muscle mass.

Other outputs include losses of protein via digestive secretions and by way of cells shed from the intestinal walls. These losses tend to be small and recouped at least in part from the large intestine, where fermentation proceeds with a microflora not unlike that of the rumen. Protein residues are digested to ammonia and absorbed as urea for reclamation in the urea cycle.

A special position applies to problems associated with parasitism. Blood sucking ectoparasites such as ticks and lice can give rise to loss of blood protein and anaemia. The same applies to flukes and roundworms which cause considerable loss of blood from the liver or the gastrointestinal mucosa. The deleterious effects of these losses may not be noticeable until the demands of production become critical as in rapidly growing calves or in potentially high-producing dairy cattle.

Problems of protein deficiency

Introduction

Protein deficiency occurs generally as a typical production disease due to imbalance between the input and output of protein supplies. Whilst meagre dietary intakes serve the needs of wild and non-productive cattle, the imposition of heavy yields of milk or rapid growth creates new problems. Furthermore, protein deficiency seldom exists as an isolated problem but usually involves other nutrients such as energy. The reasons for this can be complex. A low protein input depresses the activity of the ruminal micro-organisms so that carbohydrate digestion in the rumen fails.

Similarly, a diet poor in carbohydrate deprives the microflora of an important raw material for their multiplication and function; carbohydrate molecules, apart from supplying energy, form important templates for amino acid synthesis. Thus a deficiency of energy intake can result secondarily in protein deficiency. In addition, certain trace elements are vital for successful rumen function, including sulphur (for lysine and methionine synthesis) and cobalt. In other words, it is difficult to separate the outcome of simple protein deficiency from that of malnutrition in general.

The cause

In practice it is difficult to devise a ration truly deficient in dietary protein for the nutritional maintenance of cattle, except experimentally. Also, the additional burden of lactation is necessary to reveal the signs of a true deficiency. Dairy cows fed 75% of requirement still milk satisfactorily but suffer falls in blood urea nitrogen, and eventually in haemoglobin and albumin, which probably indicates that catabolism of protein in body tissues is being called upon to compensate for the negative balance. Some cows possess greater powers of adaptation to this negative balance than others, but in general all lactating cows give priority to the metabolic demands of the udder and use their own flesh to make good any protein deficiency.

Experimental diets, well below dietary standards for protein, lead to a decline in milk yield and milk protein content. A critical level for this to happen seems to occur when the crude protein component of the diet falls below 15% on a dry matter basis, and then only in cows giving more than 20 kg milk/day.

Has low protein intake any detrimental effects on the health of the cow? Reference has already been made to the potential danger of long-term deterioration in muscle structure and this needs further investigation to establish the true extent of this hazard. In the short term, decline in blood proteins leads to changed osmolarity of blood plasma and disorders of water metabolism with the result that oedema occurs. Also, a decline in protein synthesis may affect the production of the protein hormones connected with reproduction. If this involves reduction in the secretion of follicle stimulating hormone and luteinizing hormone then anoestrus and infertility could be expected. Another known hazard is that low protein status interferes with the synthesis of bone matrix or osteoid and that this leads to osteoporosis. Indeed, bone disorders have developed in dairy cattle fed adequate minerals and deficient only in protein. Similar disorders occur in the growth of horn leading to lameness and lesions of the hoof. Wound healing and hair growth become deleteriously affected.

The effects of protein deficiency extend to energy metabolism. The importance of proteins for the ruminal flora has received mention already and it is well known that in time of protein deficiency rumen fermentation gradually fails, as revealed by inappetance and a tendency to ruminal stasis. Energy metabolism is adversely affected also because up to 20% of blood glucose comes from the glucogenic amino acids such as alanine. In addition, methionine has a vital role in the synthesis of lipoproteins and thus any shortage of this affects fat metabolism and transport—hence protein-deficient cows may show increased susceptibility to fatty liver and ketosis.

Other diseases interact causing severe secondary protein deficiency when the cattle are fed an apparently adequate protein intake. Certain diseases of the liver and intestines lead to excessive leaking of serum protein—typical conditions of this kind include liver fluke, Johne's disease and intestinal roundworm infestations such as ostertagiasis.

Young animals show the effects of protein deficiency more than adults. They may lack the amino acids necessary for growth of new bone and muscle and hence fail to thrive, sometimes for no obvious reason. An additional factor in young animals is that they become liable to neonatal diarrhoea if they have not achieved full immunological competence from the ingestion of colostrum. Lack of proper digestion and absorption of food makes them suffer from a negative protein balance because they must break down body tissues to provide for their energy needs.

Clinical signs and diagnosis

Relatively non-specific signs predominate in protein deficiency. These include ill-thrift with stunted growth, poor quality of hair, wool or horn and a tendency to oedema. Definitive diagnosis depends on a full interpretation of a profile blood test. In the short term, protein-deficient animals always show a low blood urea concentration of less then 10.0 mg N/100 ml. In the long term this may be linked with low serum albumin (below 27 g/l) and low haemoglobin (below 10 g/100 ml), especially in lactating cows.

Differential diagnosis depends on excluding secondary effects of other deficiencies such as those of energy and trace elements, and also interaction with diseases such as parasitic infestation or Johne's disease.

Prevention and treatment

Prevention depends on a proper appreciation of the real or true intake of protein. The clinician may be misled in supposing that there is an adequate intake if he bases his conclusion solely on crude protein (or nitrogen) content. Some proteins are highly degradable in the rumen and may be inefficiently used—even simple urea appears as part of the crude protein component when based on the determination of nitrogen content.

Effective prevention and treatment follows rapidly on the correction of the dietary deficiency.

Thiamine deficiency

Introduction

A specific type of amino acid deficiency occurs in relation to a disease known as cerebrocortical necrosis or polioencephalomalacia. This occurs only sporadically but with severe, even alarming, clinical signs of nervous disorder. It is most common in young cattle fed generously on concentrates, often with minimal quantities of roughage, though it can also occur in pastured cattle when they are moved from poor to good grazing. Sometimes outbreaks occur with 25% of animals affected and with high mortality.

The cause

It is generally accepted that the cause is a specific deficiency of the amino acid thiamine. However, this is not a dietary deficiency but secondary to high levels of the enzyme thiaminase formed in the rumen, which inactivates thiamine synthesized by the rumen bacteria. The circumstances which allow this accumulation of thiaminase remain unknown. The disease can be triggered experimentally by dosing with amprolium and some other thiamine antagonists.

Clinical signs and diagnosis

Although many animals may be affected subclinically, those progressing to clinical signs suddenly become dull, difficult to handle and with unusual behaviour such as pressing their heads against walls or fences. Later they stagger, sway and then fall over with their heads drawn back in convulsive spasms. They may go blind. Most untreated animals die within a few hours, especially if young, but adults can survive for a few days or even recover with prompt treatment.

The brain lesions are typical with diffuse cerebral oedema. Histologically, there is widespread cerebral necrosis, the extent varying with the severity of clinical signs.

Diagnosis may be firmly established by measurement of the erythrocyte transketolase activity (a thiamine-dependent enzyme). Also, as thiamine controls carbohydrate metabolism, there may be elevated pyruvate and lactate concentrations in the blood. As might be expected tissue levels of thiamine are low.

Several diseases produce clinical signs resembling cerebrocortical necrosis. These include lead poisoning, hypovitaminosis A, hypomagnesaemia, brain tumours or abscesses and enterotoxaemia. Diagnosis therefore depends on excluding these other conditions.

Prevention and treatment

The only rational means of prevention seems to be to ensure an adequate intake of thiamine. A dose of 3 mg/kg of feed has been recommended but as the disease involves the destruction of thiamine by ruminal thiaminase the long-term success of this remains in doubt. On farms where the disease recurs at frequent intervals the erythrocyte transketolase test may give early warning of new cases so that intramuscular thiamine can be given with beneficial effect.

Treatment tends to be ineffective in cases showing advanced clinical signs. The usual procedure is to give thiamine intramuscularly and to monitor the response. If the animals do not return to normal in 2 days, then slaughter to salvage the carcase may be the only advisable option.

Problems of protein excess—ammonia poisoning

Introduction

The realization that urea could be used as a cheap protein supplement or replacement in ruminant diets suggested that it might find a routine place as a simple feed additive. The principle behind this idea is that rumen bacteria degrade the urea into ammonia which they then build up into amino acids and eventually into bacterial proteins. Theoretically, ruminants can use urea as a replacement for all their dietary protein, but in practice there are disadvantages. In particular, there is a danger of ammonia poisoning should the animals consume excess.

The cause

Rumen bacteria have very active urease ability for hydrolysing urea into ammonia. The problem is that they carry out this reaction much faster than they can take up the ammonia that is liberated. The excess ammonia crosses the rumen wall where it is at least partially detoxified by incorporation into glutamic acid. However, should this first detoxification mechanism be overwhelmed the ammonia proceeds to the liver, where it is dealt with by metabolism in the tricarboxylic acid cycle. Should the excess ammonia reach the systemic circulation then toxic effects ensue in the central nervous system. It is estimated that toxicity occurs when excess rumen ammonia exceeds 176 mg/100 ml and when blood ammonia rises above 1–4 mg/100 ml. Toxic doses of urea seem to lie between 0.31–0.44 g/kg body weight depending on nutritional status and adaptation of the animal to a steady intake of urea.

Various predisposing factors operate. A sudden intake of urea is much more dangerous than a long-term and steady input. Also, animals are highly susceptible if their diet is deficient in fermentable carbohydrate or if they are semi-starved. A sufficient substrate

of carbohydrate molecules seems to be highly protective in promoting maximum uptake of ammonia by the ruminal bacteria.

Clinical signs and diagnosis

Clinical signs originate from the derangement of the central
nervous system. The animals become uneasy and dull. Soon
muscle tremors start with excess salivation, rapid respiration and
incoordination, tetany and death. Tremors and spasms of muscles
seem to be an important diagnostic sign.

Post-mortem examination reveals evidence of circulatory collapse and venous stasis. Epicardial and endocardial haemorrhages
can be found together with pulmonary oedema and haemorrhage.

Several tissues accumulate ammonia—especially muscle—and
ammonia concentration in these as well as in the blood is diagnostic. Blood urea is commonly very high.

Prevention and treatment

An important principle is to introduce urea very slowly and
cautiously into a new diet. Unfortunately, urea supplements tend
to be reserved for animals in poor nutritional state when they will
be eager for food of any kind and their tolerance to urea will be at its
lowest. Thus dominant cattle will ravenously eat more than their
share and die leaving others to follow in a similar way. This
inequality of intake can be fatal; the calculated, safe amount of urea
which should be inocuous if consumed equally by all the stock,
becomes dangerous if the aggressive animals consume the most.
Thus good management is the most effective preventive.

Treatment of urea toxicity is an emergency procedure. Massive
doses of acetic acid may be effective (i.e. 18 litres of 5% acetic acid
to alleviate the immediate clinical signs), but it must be given very
early in the disease process. A radical expedient is to remove the
rumen contents by rumenotomy.

8/Trace element deficiencies

Iodine

Introduction

The obvious outcome of iodine deficiency is enlargement of the thyroid gland or goitre, especially in newborn calves. However, many of the effects remain insidious involving non-specific reduction in metabolism and productive capacity, together with a high incidence of abortion, stillbirth and calf mortality. Deficiency is widespread. Most roughage intakes of cattle tend to be deficient in iodine for their needs. This is made worse by interacting factors such as high intakes of calcium which limit iodine absorption, and also certain *Brassica* species of plants, containing cyanogenetic glucosides, which are capable of inducing goitre in areas of marginal iodine deficiency. Furthermore, inland areas tend to become increasingly deficient because supplies are gradually removed by the grazing livestock without replacement. There is the added complication that some grass species (e.g. Yorkshire fog) contain less iodine than others.

The cause

Nearly all of the iodine in the body is stored in the thyroid gland in the form of thyroglobulin or thyroxine. In fact, iodine has no physiological function on its own but is a component of the thyroid hormones. These exert important functions controlling energy exchange and metabolic rate, together with tissue growth.

Iodine deficiency leads to goitre because decreased secretion of thyroxine by the thyroid gland stimulates the pituitary to secrete thyrotropic hormone which in turn induces enlargement of the thyroid, hopefully to produce more hormone—an impossibility if iodine deficiency is the limiting factor and hence progressive increase in size of the thyroid gland ensues. Deficiency of thyroxine has other effects. Animals lack energy, show progressive weakness, and often appear hairless because of decrease in the thickness of the hair follicles.

91

The simple effect of iodine deficiency is made worse by the presence of thiocyanates which depress iodine uptake by the thyroid. These compounds can originate from many plants which contain cyanogenetic glucosides (e.g. kale) which on conversion into thiocyanate become goiterogenic, especially in areas where subclinical iodine deficiency already exists.

Clinical signs and diagnosis

A general decline in basal metabolism leads to a wide range of non-specific clinical signs. These include failure to thrive, disappointing milk yield and general debility. There will also be a general decline in sexual drive and function. A more specific diagnostic sign is a high incidence of abortion and stillbirth, with several of the dead calves showing goitre. This may or may not be accompanied by lack of hair covering.

Precise diagnosis depends on analysis of the iodine content of blood, urine, or even milk. However, the interpretation of these tests requires care because iodine deficiency is a long-term problem, the thyroid gland storing sufficient to tide the animal over for long periods. Concentrate rations usually contain ample iodine so that it may only be during the grazing season when deficiency gradually prevails and the animals show a protracted decline in blood or milk iodine. Surveys reveal that many herds show milk iodine levels below a critical value of 20 μg/l, yet few of these seem to suffer overt ill effects. Conversely, many herds show surprisingly high levels of milk iodine—a spurious result probably due to the use of iodine in teat dips which contaminate the milk samples.

Blood tests are more appropriate for diagnosis of iodine deficiency in non-lactating cattle, plasma iodine, either total or protein bound, being satisfactory (levels below 2.0 μg/100 ml are diagnostic). Alternatively plasma thyroxine has been used.

Prevention and treatment

The simple correction of the dietary deficiency should be sufficient once the diagnosis has been made. Most compound feedingstuffs contain adequate supplies though iodized salt blocks should be provided for stock grazing outdoors. Recommendations suggest that an iodine intake of 1 mg/kg of dry matter of feed is enough for lactating cows, or 0.1 mg/kg for non-lactating cows or calves.

Over-zealous supplementation induces the clinical problem of iodine excess or iodism. Fortunately, only very high and continuous dosage induces this, excess iodine being excreted in the urine and milk. Even so, 160 mg/day becomes toxic for cows, with proportionately less for calves. Signs of toxicity include failure to eat, hyperexcitability and a tendency to hyperthermia. The skin becomes affected, with loss of coat condition and hair.

Iron

Introduction

Iron occurs plentifully on most pastures so that deficiency in grazing animals rarely exists. However, milk-fed calves commonly suffer from it because milk is a poor source of iron and the newborn calf possesses only sufficient reserves for 2–3 weeks. Most of the iron in the body occurs in the haemoglobin of the red blood cells, or in the myoglobin of muscle. Thus iron deficiency inevitably leads to anaemia.

The cause

Iron deficiency anaemia occurs most commonly in intensively reared calves intended for veal. The important factor is that these animals feed almost entirely on milk or milk substitutes which have a low content of iron. To a certain extent this situation is planned because consumers expect that veal be relatively pale in colour and thus a certain degree of anaemia is desirable. However, this carries a penalty because anaemia leads to poor growth and protein conversion; hence the feeding of veal calves needs careful management so that the flesh remains pale but without sufficient anaemia to interfere seriously with productivity. Deleterious effects of anaemia seem to occur when haemoglobin levels in the blood fall below 8 g/100 ml. Additional untoward effects in anaemic calves include a higher than normal incidence of infectious diseases, especially of diarrhoea and pneumonia.

A surprisingly high incidence of anaemia is present in milk-fed calves—surveys revealing as much as 13–35%—predictable because calves need 50 mg of iron daily, but a milk diet contains only 2–4 mg.

Anaemia also occurs in adult cattle but this is seldom linked with iron deficiency. More common causes include loss of haemoglobin in post-parturient haemoglobinuria, in parasitic infestations, or as a result of kale toxicity. Anaemia due to actual iron deficiency, said to respond to supplementation, may appear in housed bulls or growing stock fed severely limited or inadequate diets, when several factors may be involved.

Clinical signs and diagnosis

Subclinical anaemia may induce non-specific effects such as poor growth rate and a high incidence of infectious disease. Loss of appetite provides the most sensitive indicator of early anaemia. However, more severe anaemia can be identified by the pallor of mucous membranes and paleness of the blood. Liver degeneration with yellowing due to fatty change may be seen in dead animals.

The most effective diagnostic method involves blood tests for evidence of anaemia, either by haematocrit determination or haemoglobin assay. An haematocrit of less than 26% or haemoglobin below 8 g/100 ml are critical levels at which iron supplementation should become beneficial.

Prevention and treatment

The most effective prevention and treatment for anaemia in calves is dietary supplementation with iron. Between 25–30 mg Fe/kg feed dry matter should suffice without spoiling the desired pale appearance of the veal. However, even higher doses may yield an additional growth response.

Copper

Introduction

Copper deficiency occurs widely. This follows not only from a simple deficiency of copper, but also because of interaction with other trace elements such as molybdenum and possibly also of iron and sulphur. Copper plays an important part in tissue oxidation, especially in relation to the cytochrome oxidase system, failure of which leads to a wide variety of clinical problems.

The cause

Soils in many parts of the world show a primary deficiency of copper for grazing stock. However, this is exacerbated should the deficiency be combined with an excess of molybdenum. Only 10 ppm of molybdenum interferes with copper absorption and converts a marginal deficiency into a major problem. Secondary deficiencies of this kind are especially prone to occur on soils where the underlying rock is composed of molybdenum-rich shales. The situation is made more complex by the relatively common occurrence of concurrent deficiencies of both copper, cobalt and possibly also of selenium.

Excess sulphur also limits copper absorption. The sulphur need not be inorganic in origin, but organic in the form of sulphur-containing amino acids such as lysine and methionine, which are present in abundance in protein-rich diets. It is believed that the sulphur converts the copper into insoluble copper sulphide which resists absorption. Excess calcium also inhibits absorption of copper. Hence fresh liming of pasture may precipitate an unexpected outbreak of copper deficiency.

As a general rule, pasture containing less than 3 ppm dry matter of copper initiates clinical signs of copper deficiency but the presence of molybdenum or other interacting factors makes the situation worse—with very high intakes of molybdenum even generous copper supplementation proves inadequate. A ratio of Cu:Mo of 5:1 may be optimal. Fortunately, concentrate rations usually contain enough copper so that deficiency seldom develops in housed animals receiving supplementary feeds, though of course this favourable position does not apply to indoor stock receiving only silage grown on deficient pasture.

The cause of the many lesions of copper deficiency stems from faulty oxidative metabolism in tissues. This leads to loss of body condition and failure to thrive. Similarly, loss of function in the intestinal villi leads to failure of absorption and the diarrhoea which is a characteristic feature of copper deficiency, and depression of osteoblast metabolism in bones leads to defective growth and osteoporosis.

Anaemia is another consequence. This is due to the involvement of copper in haemoglobin synthesis, especially in the re-use of haemosiderin, a breakdown product of haemoglobin. The effect of copper deficiency in causing loss of hair colour follows from inadequate oxidation of thiol groups as the hair becomes keratinized in the follicles. The myocardial degeneration and ventricular fibrillation which can cause sudden death in copper-deficient cattle may be due to impairment of tissue oxidation in the heart wall. Finally, defective myelinization may follow from inhibited oxidation in the neurones, which comes into play during fetal life.

Clinical signs and diagnosis

As mentioned above, a wide variety of clinical signs link with copper deficiency. Early signs are non-specific and include poor growth (so-called 'pine') and roughness of hair coat with loss of pigmentation. Later, diarrhoea (especially on 'teart' or molybdenum-rich pastures) together with lameness and abnormalities of limb bones make their appearance. Anaemia also develops progressively. Most of these changes come on slowly over several months because the liver possesses a large copper storage capacity and maintains blood levels for long periods.

In some cases copper deficiency provokes sudden death. This clinical sign is known as 'falling disease'. Affected animals suddenly bellow, collapse and die, presumably from a direct derangement of myocardial function.

Definitive diagnosis of copper deficiency presents problems partly because it often coexists with cobalt or selenium deficiency. In many cases a survey of the trace element status of the soils and plants may be advisable. Indeed, exhaustive surveys have been carried out over whole regions or complete countries, but results need careful interpretation. 'Clinically silent' hypocuprosis is common and there is no guarantee that copper supplementation will benefit such herds. Indeed, hypocupraemia is surprisingly common, sometimes affecting half the herds surveyed, though most improve performance on supplementation. Blood copper levels below 0.05 mg/l are usually considered to be diagnostic.

Although blood samples appear to be the medium of choice in diagnosis of copper deficiency, many consider that liver copper gives a better indication. Unfortunately, this means that liver biopsies must be obtained, or that abattoir specimens must be sought. Other options include hair and milk. Although several investigators have found close correlations between all these methods several factors must be taken into account. First, at best, hair only reflects copper levels retrospectively relevant to the time of hair growth, and great care is needed to wash the hairs thoroughly to clean them from faecal contamination. Second, hair copper levels vary with factors such as hair colour—white hair is said to show more promise as an indicator. Third, liver copper values gauge the level of copper reserves remaining in the liver, blood levels remaining held until liver copper runs out, say below 20 mg/l.

Two alternatives exist for screening blood copper. Caeruloplasmin concentration has advantages, correlating very closely with blood copper and being easier to analyse. Others consider the erythrocyte superoxide dismutase test to have value.

Prevention and treatment

The usual recommendation is to ensure that the diet of cattle has a copper content of about 10 mg/kg of food on a dry matter basis. However, this is not always practicable for animals on pasture. Oral doses of copper sulphate (about 4 g) may help, though mineral mixtures may be easier to allow on free access. Top dressings to pasture also prove effective (5–6 kg/ha copper sulphate).

All methods of supplementation need careful supervision because of the danger of copper poisoning. Cattle are less liable to suffer toxic effects of over-dosage than sheep, but even so a dose of 220–880 mg/kg body weight can prove fatal. Chronic poisoning may occur if the pasture exceeds 15–20 mg/kg dry matter, depending on the molybdenum content which serves to give a protective effect.

Probably a safer and more accurate way of supplementation is to give copper by parenteral injection. Several preparations exist which release copper gradually giving cover for several months and also avoiding the inhibitory effect of molybdenum on intestinal absorption. In addition, the timing of the injection can be arranged to maximum advantage. A good time is shortly before parturition so that the newborn calf will have built up its reserves *in utero* and the mother will have received sufficient herself to prevent infertility.

Cobalt

Introduction

Cobalt deficiency certainly occurs in many parts of the world but we lack precise knowledge about it simply because there is no easy and reliable indicator of cobalt status in the animal. Doubtless cobalt deficiency limits growth and causes wasting—the problem is the lack of a good diagnostic test to define the extent of the problem.

The cause

Large areas of pasture are cobalt deficient for grazing cattle, primarily because of a simple deficiency of cobalt in the soil. Deficiency probably exists when the soil contains less than 0.25 ppm cobalt. However, the situation becomes complex when it is realized that several interactions limit the availability of cobalt to the plants and the grazing animals. For example, uptake into plants varies inversely with soil pH. Hence, alkaline soils or heavy dressings with lime depress cobalt levels in the forage. Also, some new and improved strains of grass contain a low cobalt content. This is why improvements in pasture management may trigger clinical deficiency in a hitherto marginal situation.

Cobalt is only of value to the animal because it is part of the structure of the vitamin B_{12} molecule which is an essential vitamin serving as an activator for several enzyme systems connected with energy metabolism. Vitamin B_{12} also plays a key role in the generation of red blood cells. In more detail, the deficient animal suffers curtailment in the metabolism of propionic acid, methylmalonic and succinic acids. Also, affected animals become anaemic. In practical terms this means that cobalt deficiency leads to a wide variety of deleterious effects such as low production, either of growth or milk, poor appetite together with infertility and ketosis. The main cause of these changes comes from an impaired ability to metabolize propionate and synthesize glucose.

Ruminants are fortunate in that ample supplies of vitamin B_{12}

can be synthesized by the ruminal micro-organisms, but only if sufficient cobalt is available. The vitamin thus formed is readily absorbed across the rumen wall.

Clinical signs and diagnosis

No specific signs denote cobalt deficiency. The most obvious general effect is a gradual decrease in appetite with loss of body weight. Some cattle show pica. Diarrhoea and severe wasting supervene later as the deficiency progresses.

Diagnosis presents difficulties because there is no simple test yet perfected to reveal the deficient animal or farm. Determination of cobalt in blood plasma may be attempted but vitamin B_{12} assay is more usual. At one time this involved cumbersome bioassays based on the growth of vitamin B_{12}-requiring bacteria. More recently, radioassay methods have received favour. In spite of these difficulties, surveys of vitamin B_{12} status have identified herds capable of responding to cobalt supplementation. Few reliable standards denote deficiency. In general, normal levels of vitamin B_{12} lie in the range 300–400 $\mu g/ml$ blood plasma, with less than 250 $\mu g/ml$ indicating deficiency.

An important complicating factor is that reserves of vitamin B_{12} are laid down in the liver providing cover for up to 5 weeks. Thus some investigators consider liver vitamin B_{12} a more reliable test, levels of 0.3 $\mu g/g$ liver being enough to support optimum growth, but 0.1 $\mu g/g$ being liable to lead to clinical signs.

Yet another alternative test involves estimation of methylmalonic acid in the urine. This acid is usually metabolized in a vitamin B_{12} enzyme system, but in cobalt-deficient animals it escapes metabolism to be excreted via the kidneys. Another, similar compound escaping metabolism in vitamin B_{12} deficiency is formiminoglutamic acid. Relatively high levels of this in the urine also denote vitamin B_{12} deficiency. This is the basis of the so-called FIGLU test. Both tests require cautious interpretation.

Although not specific diagnostically, affected animals often show anaemia and hypoglycaemia. These changes taken into account with other clinical signs may help the clinician come to a firm diagnosis.

Prevention and treatment

An important point is that cobalt supplementation must be given orally to be effective, otherwise it will not be converted into vitamin B_{12} by the ruminal bacteria. Parenteral injections of cobalt have little benefit, although preformed vitamin B_{12} may be given directly by this route.

Recommended levels of cobalt in the diet are 0.07 mg/kg dry matter. This can be achieved in deficient areas if cobalt sulphate is used as a pasture dressing (400–600 g/ha) its value persisting for some 3–4 years. Alternatively, a wide range of pellets, bullets or glass boluses have been devised for intraruminal administration. Finally, an intramuscular injection of vitamin B_{12} may be given which, although costly, confers immediate effect lasting throughout the grazing season.

Overdosing with cobalt rarely occurs. Toxic signs have been recorded in calves receiving food containing 40–55 mg of cobalt/50 kg body weight, well over the recommended dose. The signs included failure to eat, rough coat, listlessness and incoordination.

Selenium

Introduction

Selenium deficiency recently assumed prominence as an important and widespread problem. Much of this new interest stemmed, first, from our knowledge of selenium's role in cell metabolism and, second, from the fact that a reliable and simple diagnostic test became available for use in diagnosis and surveys.

Together with vitamin E, selenium protects cell membranes against the toxic action of certain lipid peroxides. In other words, both vitamin E and selenium act as antioxidants. Selenium works in this way because it is a component of the enzyme glutathione peroxidase. Hence, deficiency of selenium leads to shortage of the enzyme which in turn allows the accumulation of toxic peroxides. On the other hand, vitamin E acts not so much as an antioxidant but as a limiting factor in the conversion of unsaturated fatty acids to lipid peroxides. Thus both exert a parallel and protective function. Many selenium-responsive diseases respond equally well to vitamin E and vice versa.

The cause

The soils of several parts of the world are deficient in selenium. In general, soils from sedimentary rocks contain more selenium than those derived from igneous rocks. Acidic soils also tend to be deficient and the low pH inhibits the uptake of selenium into plants. Furthermore, as might be expected, plants growing in low selenium soils tend to contain little selenium in their leaves, acidity merely worsening the situation. A selenium concentration in plants of below 0.1 ppm is accepted as the critical level at which clinical signs begin to occur. In one survey of the UK 47% of farms were relatively deficient and the grazing livestock were presumably at risk.

Selenium deficiency becomes especially important if there is a coincidental deficiency of vitamin E. Inferior hay or straw contains relatively little vitamin E. Also, certain methods of storing and preserving moist grains, e.g. with propionic acid, destroy the vitamin E content. Even without preservative moist grain loses its vitamin E content in about 6 months and will allow clinical signs to occur if it is fed alongside a selenium-deficient forage.

Vitamin E and selenium deficiency lead to so-called 'nutritional or enzootic muscular dystrophy'. The cause of this, as described above, is a failure to prevent the accumulation of toxic peroxides on cell membranes. Sometimes an additional precipitating factor operates. For instance, unsaturated fatty acids in fish or vegetable oils seem to function as myopathic agents, presumably overwhelming the function of limited supplies of vitamin E. Also, unaccustomed muscular exercise may trigger the breakdown and necrosis of muscle fibres which already have accumulated toxic levels of peroxides.

The lesions of muscular dystrophy occur mainly in young, rapidly growing calves. Clinical signs commonly appear when they are turned out to grass in the spring. Many may die, sudden deaths being commonly due to lesions in the muscles of the heart wall (myocardial dystrophy) alongside those in the main skeletal muscles.

A non-specific, less acute form of the disease occurs, the main clinical sign being ill-thrift. Even so, the loss of production with poor growth and diarrhoea, which this condition causes, can result in severe economic loss. Other non-specific effects are said to include a high incidence of retained fetal membranes, but its relationship to selenium deficiency remains obscure, though it is said to respond to selenium supplementation.

Clinical signs and diagnosis

An attack of nutritional muscular dystrophy presents alarming signs. Affected calves suddenly collapse and cannot rise. Even when supported they refuse to bear weight. Rapid pulse and respiration rates are typical, coupled with heart irregularities when lesions damage the heart wall. Frequently, more than one calf is affected simultaneously and an association with unusual exercise or turnout to pasture may be noted as a common factor. If the disease comes on gradually there may be warning signs of stiffness and reluctance to rise.

At post-mortem examination large segments of muscle appear abnormally pale or even white. Often the lesions lie in streaks following the lines of the muscle fibres. The dead muscle eventually calcifies and undergoes fibrosis. In cases where the heart is involved the white lesions of muscle degeneration appear under the lining of the left ventricle, extending into the septum. Again the damaged muscle eventually calcifies. Histologically, the affected muscles suffer coagulative necrosis showing a hyaline homogeneous appearance as compared with the normal adjacent fibres.

Several clinical tests confirm diagnosis. Enzyme leakage from the damaged muscle fibres into the blood is an important indicator, the concentration of enzyme giving a measure of the extent of the muscle lesions. Plasma creatine phosphokinase (CPK) is highly specific for both cardiac and skeletal muscle. Normally the levels of CPK are low (about 20–30 IU/l) but soar to above 1000 or even 10 000 IU/l in the blood of severe cases. In survivors the levels return to normal after a few days, unless the lesions become progressive and hence the test must be carried out promptly. Other muscle enzymes which can be measured for the same purpose include serum glutamic oxalo transaminase (GOT). Alternatively, some investigators prefer to measure the level of a breakdown product of muscle metabolism, creatine, in the urine.

In many instances, however, the clinician will wish to monitor the actual selenium status of animals on a farm to predict the possibility of an outbreak. Dietary selenium may be measured—about 0.1 ppm is adequate. Tissue levels of selenium may be helpful also if abattoir specimens are available. Blood and milk levels have been used. Adequate blood selenium usually amounts to 0.10 μg/ml with 0.05 μg/ml being a critical point for diagnosis of deficiency. Although blood selenium measures selenium status directly, many use the selenium-containing enzyme, glutathione peroxidase of erythrocytes, as a practical alternative. Levels of glutathione peroxidase below 200 mU/l of blood are thought to indicate selenium deficiency.

Blood selenium and glutathione peroxidase estimations provide especially useful indicators in cases of non-specific ill-thrift, without overt muscle disease. Such cases frequently respond beneficially to selenium supplementation even when the existence of a problem may not have been suspected.

Prevention and treatment

Some difficulty is experienced because of the overlapping functions of selenium and vitamin E. In general, it is wisest to ensure the adequate provision of both. However, selenium alone may prove to be protective even in cases where vitamin E is deficient. Fortunately, selenium crosses the placenta and thus a strategic dose of selenium given to the cow in late pregnancy gives protection to both mother and her calf. The protection can be long lasting because the kidneys and liver store reserves. Alternatively, selenium may be given in the feed—about 0.1 ppm is thought to be satisfactory. Mineral supplements containing selenium may also be offered. In cases of doubt the blood glutathione peroxidase test can be used as a monitoring test.

Prophylactic and therapeutic injections of selenium have been used. A generally recommended dose is 0.1 mg/kg body weight, which should maintain the selenium status of an animal for up to 6 months. However, extreme care is needed in computing the dose because selenium is very toxic. For instance, 1 mg/kg body weight can kill; admittedly ten times the therapeutic level but decimal points can be misplaced. It is also important not to confuse the dosage of selenium with that for anhydrous sodium selenite or sodium selenate—the above doses refer to selenium in its elemental form. The manufacturer's instructions must be carefully obeyed.

Zinc

Introduction

Realization of the importance of zinc deficiency followed recent advances in our understanding of zinc metabolism. A wide group of defects link with it including poor growth, slow healing of wounds, infertility and impaired immunological competence with low resistance to infection. Zinc is a molecular component of various enzymes, or polymerases, which synthesize DNA and RNA and thus any body function dependent on the replication of cells or the synthesis of proteins will be affected by zinc deficiency.

The cause

Perhaps surprisingly zinc metabolism receives good homeostatic control. Efficiency of absorption rises to nearly 100% in times of deficiency. Also, endogenous excretion into the faeces and output into the milk can be drastically restricted. Furthermore, a storage mechanism exists with good reserves of zinc laid down in the liver and bones. This tends to circumvent the effects of temporary deficiency. Another important factor is that zinc deficiency need not be due solely to a simple low intake because there is strong interaction for absorption with calcium, iron and copper.

Zinc circulates in the blood in either free or protein bound forms though most tests for nutritional adequacy rely on the measurement of total zinc concentration.

Mention was made above that zinc is a component of several enzymes related to protein synthesis and cell division. This explains its involvement with immunocompetence and resistance to infectious disease because it is associated with the production of immunoglobulin proteins and with the generation of blood cells such as polymorphs and lymphocytes. A further characteristic effect of zinc deficiency follows from its involvement with cell replication in the skin. The interruption in the orderly growth of epidermal cells leads to inflammation or dermatitis and parakeratosis which occurs typically on the hind limbs, udder and teats. This means that the skin of the teats ulcerates easily, even with the mild trauma of milking. Similarly, the growth of horn becomes disordered leading to lesions of the hooves and persistent lameness.

Finally, impairment of cell replication and protein synthesis leads to ill-thrift and failure to grow. The skeleton is particularly affected because the growth plates at the ends of long bones show inactivity and the protein matrix fails to provide a good framework for mineralization.

One unusual cause of zinc deficiency involves an inherited or congenital disease of certain strains of cattle which develop parakeratosis even on apparently normal intakes of zinc. A defect in zinc absorption has been proposed.

Clinical signs and diagnosis

The main clinical sign is parakeratosis of the skin accompanied by hairlessness (alopecia). Stunted growth, stiffness and swelling of the coronets above the feet are also seen. Particularly characteristic features include wrinkling and cracking of the skin on the knees and hocks. Also there is a pronounced delay in the healing of wounds.

Histologically, the skin lesion of parakeratosis, though characteristic, is not entirely diagnostic. Most investigators depend on measuring the concentration of total zinc in the blood serum. Nutritional intake predominates in controlling this—in fact, serum zinc responds rapidly to a zinc-deficient diet, a fall of 50% within 1 week being typical. Problems of interpretation need full appreciation. First, great care is needed to avoid zinc contamination of all the glassware used for blood sampling. Second, the precise meaning of the concentration remains in doubt; levels of zinc now classified as normal may not be truly optimal for healthy growth and productivity. Present understanding is that the normal lies between 80–120 μg/100 ml serum with a provisional threshold for deficiency at 70 μg/100 ml serum.

An alternative indicator of zinc status is metallothionein, a metabolite containing zinc which is synthesized in the liver. It is thought that this gives an improved measure of the zinc reserves remaining in the liver as opposed to the immediate input.

Some investigators recommend hair as the sample medium for zinc assessment. However, this is not always reliable because very large changes in diet are needed to show altered concentrations.

Prevention and treatment

Prevention depends on ensuring an adequate dietary intake of zinc. Concentrate rations usually contain sufficient. Care must be taken to avoid over-zealous supplementation but cases of toxicity rarely occur, probably because cattle reduce absorption from the diet if they eat zinc to excess. Satisfactory values for zinc in feed are recommended as 40 ppm dry matter for calves though higher levels (90 ppm) are said to be appropriate for grazing cattle. It is surprising that zinc deficiency occurs at all due to the general use of galvanized pipes and tanks for water distribution.

Manganese

Introduction

Manganese is another trace element associated with key enzymes in metabolism. In this case they include the phosphorylating enzymes synthesizing ATP, alkaline phosphatase and pyruvate oxidase. Manganese also appears to be vital for the proper development of the genital organs.

The cause

Manganese is unique in trace element metabolism in that it is very poorly absorbed (at most about 1%) from the diet and is almost totally removed from the portal blood as it filters through the liver. This means that very low concentrations of manganese appear in the systemic circulation.

Primary deficiencies of manganese occur in some areas where there is a low concentration in local rock and soils. Also, an excess of calcium and phosphorus is said to interfere with absorption. A critical level for deficiency appears to be below 3 ppm, but heavy dressings of lime and high pH may mean that a higher concentration could be desirable in certain circumstances. Pasture herbage containing less than 80 ppm may not be enough to support normal fertility.

Manganese is active in forming the matrix of bone and cartilage. Hence lameness and skeletal abnormalities ensue in deficiency.

Newborn calves suffer from congenital deformation of the limbs with enlarged joints and knuckling of the fetlocks.

Infertility is another common event with delay coming into oestrus, failure to conceive, and small underdeveloped ovaries.

Clinical signs and diagnosis

Limb deformities in calves and infertility in cows are predominant signs. Blood analysis is seldom undertaken because of the very low levels of manganese occurring normally in the systemic circulation. Possibly the only remaining alternative is to assess the potential value of a dietary supplement of manganese—in other words an empirical 'try it and see' test.

Prevention and treatment

Cattle may show an improvement in fertility to a supplement of 2 g $MnSO_4$ daily. More can be fed without danger because the cow absorbs so little. It is said that massive supplementation, up to 5 000 ppm in the diet, reduces appetite and weight gain.

9/Vitamin deficiencies

Vitamin A

Introduction

Deficiency of vitamin A should occur only rarely in cattle. This is because all green plants on the pasture contain abundant supplies of the vitamin A precursor, carotene. However, certain kinds of modern husbandry entail that cattle do not always have access, especially if they are housed and fed conserved forage with supplements such as roots or sugar beet pulp which do not contain vitamin A. Fortunately, the clinical signs of deficiency are easily recognized and are therefore readily corrected. The signs include skin disease, blindness, abnormal growth of the skeleton and infertility.

The cause

Cattle receive vitamin A either preformed as an additive to their concentrate ration, or as the precursor carotene. Carotene is a yellow pigment found in the leaves of nearly all pasture plants. On ingestion the intestinal wall converts it to vitamin A, though much of the carotene enters the systemic circulation without conversion.

Unfortunately, carotene is destroyed by drying and bleaching in the sun as happens during the making of hay or when the pasture becomes affected by drought. Thus cattle become deficient when fed poor-quality weathered hay, or when left to graze brown and withered fields.

Calves receive vitamin A in colostrum, usually enough to tide them over until more can be obtained from other sources. It should be noted that carotene cannot cross the placenta and thus even though the cows graze green pasture during late pregnancy the calves may be born with low reserves of vitamin A in their livers. In contrast, vitamin A can cross the placenta and thus concentrate rations containing the preformed vitamin do contribute to fetal reserves.

Several factors can induce secondary deficiency of vitamin A. These include chronic disease of the intestines which restricts the conversion of carotene. Phosphorus deficiency and high intakes of nitrate are said to have a similar effect. A special problem ensues if cattle receive continuous treatment with mineral oil to prevent bloat; the mineral oil takes up the fat-soluble carotene and the vitamin thus effectively removing it from absorption. Finally, vitamin A and carotene are easily oxidized and thus a feed which originally contained ample easily deteriorates on storage.

Clinical signs of vitamin A deficiency take a long time to develop because the liver has good storage capacity, capable of lasting for 6 or more months. However, even this reserve gives out eventually. Probably beef cows experience the main difficulty when they come off dry and brown summer pasture containing little green herbage and go into winter quarters on diets containing poor-quality roughage. In these circumstances pregnant cattle, which start the winter with low reserves, become progressively more deficient and then give birth to congenitally defective calves in the spring.

Vitamin A performs several important functions. First, it is vital for the regeneration of visual purple, a pigment essential for light receptivity in the retinal cells of the eye. Thus an initial defect caused by vitamin A deficiency is reduced sight in dim light which eventually leads to blindness. Second, the vitamin is essential for the balanced function of osteoblasts and osteoclasts in bone. These two types of cell exert opposing functions; osteoblasts lay down new bone, whereas osteoclasts resorb pre-existing bone. Disturbance of this balance distorts the bone remodelling process as growth proceeds. Failure to remodel leads to gradual occlusion of the openings or foramina of the skull and vertebral column. The nerves which emerge through these openings undergo gradual constriction and compression. Constriction of the optic nerve in this way is one of the causes of blindness associated with vitamin A deficiency, in addition to the effect on the retina described above.

Third, vitamin A deficiency upsets skin growth. The secretory cells in the sebaceous glands undergo keratinization and cease to secrete the oils which protect and confer coat condition. Also, the epidermis covering the eyeball keratinizes leading to opacity or xerophthalmia. Fourth, vitamin A is essential for the orderly development of the fetal tissues and thus deficiency leads to a variety of congenital abnormalities. Finally, vitamin A controls the resorption of cerebrospinal fluid through the arachnoid villi. Thus, in deficiency, this fluid accumulates with such increased pressure that convulsions occur and hydrocephalus commonly appears in the fetus and young calf.

Clinical signs and diagnosis

Inability to see in dim light may be the first clinical sign. Affected cattle walk into obstructions. Later total blindness ensues. The most obvious lesion causing this appears in calves as a cloudiness and thickening of the cornea of the eye, often accompanied by ulceration and infection. Also the skin becomes rough, dry and scaly. Painful cracks may develop in the hooves causing lameness.

Nervous signs occur, particularly in young calves. In part these result from constriction of the cranial and spinal nerves as they emerge from the central nervous system through the various foramina (as described above). Thus constriction of the optic nerves leads to total and irreversible blindness, whilst constriction of the spinal nerves paralyses various parts of the body depending on the distribution of the affected nerves. In addition, increased cerebrospinal fluid pressure leads to convulsions, especially and easily provoked in calves that are moved or disturbed for any reason.

Infertility is an important clinical result of vitamin A deficiency. The seminiferous tubules of the testis undergo atrophy so that bulls fail to produce semen with sufficient spermatozoa. In pregnant females placental degeneration occurs, with the birth of calves showing a high incidence of congenital defects.

Diagnosis depends on measurement of vitamin A in plasma. A normal level for optimal health is put at 25 μg/dl with clinical signs predictable at 5 μg/dl. Plasma carotene also gives a useful indication of vitamin A status. Cattle on green pasture normally have yellow plasma simply due to large amounts of carotene which may reach 150 μg/dl. Some investigators prefer to rely on the levels of vitamin A in the liver, but the measurement of this requires either liver biopsies or abattoir specimens.

Prevention and treatment

The minimum daily requirement is 40 IU of vitamin A per kg of body weight, though considerably more than this is needed for pregnant and lactating cattle. However, few clinicians rely on the simple computation of intake, realizing the many complicating circumstances. It is more usual to be aware of the situations in which deficiencies occur and supplement the diet as seems appropriate. An alternative is to give intramuscular injections of vitamin A. Given at 2 monthly intervals 3000–6000 IU/kg confers long-term cover taking advantage of the liver's storage capacity.

Parenteral injection is to be preferred for treatment purposes. A rapid response is usually achieved provided the lesions have not progressed irreversibly.

Excessive intakes of vitamin A are not normally toxic. However, very large doses (100 times normal) given experimentally induce bony exostoses and lameness. It must, however, be remembered that vitamin A acts as a vitamin D antagonist and even provokes clinical hypovitaminosis D in stock which are already marginally deficient in vitamin D. The two vitamins A and D and the two minerals calcium and phosphorus interact one with the other. Correct balance between all four ensures optimal development of bone and growth.

Vitamin D

Introduction

The dangers of a simple vitamin D deficiency are so well known, especially for calves, that supplements are usually given long before clinical signs appear. The common clinical signs are rickets in calves and osteomalacia in adults. However, recent knowledge about the complex interrelationships between the minerals calcium and phosphorus and the vitamins A and D, and possibly also with protein status, reveals an insidious subclinical situation which can cause severe loss of productivity without any obvious lesions.

The cause

Vitamin D or its precursors enter the body by three routes. The most important is by solar irradiation. Ultraviolet light converts a precursor, 7-dihydrocholesterol, in the skin to the active compound cholecalciferol. A similar type of reaction occurs when sunlight irradiates certain steroids in plants so that conserved forage such as hay serves as a source of the vitamin. Alternatively, preformed vitamin D can be added to the diet in milk, or in milk replacer feed for calves, or in concentrates for adult cattle.

Lack of ultraviolet irradiation is an important cause of vitamin D deficiency. This is especially important at increasing distance from the equator where the sun's rays become progressively weaker. Winter, overcast skies and smoky atmospheres all contribute to the problem. Also, cattle with thick or darkly-coloured coats receive little sunlight on their skin and are consequently susceptible to deficiency. Similarly, housed animals receive no direct sunlight and as these are commonly young and rapidly growing they show signs of deficiency very rapidly.

Simple deficiency of vitamin D may not be the only cause of a clinical problem. For example, an antagonist such as carotene has an antivitamin D effect. Thus calves, which are marginally deficient indoors, may suddenly succumb to rickets when turned out onto green pasture.

Vitamin D has a complex metabolism within the body. Cholecalciferol (Vitamin D_3) is produced in the skin by irradiation with ultraviolet light. However, this form of the vitamin is not immediately fully active. It needs hydroxylation in two stages. The first takes place in the liver to 25-dihydroxycholecalciferol. The second stage occurs in the kidney, either to 24,25-dihydroxycholecalciferol, or to 1,25-dihydroxycholecalciferol. The difference is important because the 24,25-form is relatively inactive and is excreted in the urine. On the other hand, the 1,25-form is preferred if the animal needs calcium and is under the stimulus of parathyroid hormone. This final, fully hydroxylated vitamin initiates the intestinal absorption of calcium and the mineralization of bone. Thus vitamin D exerts a complex role as part of an endocrinological sequence in the control of calcium metabolism.

Clinically, the most important effect of vitamin D deficiency is defective growth and mineralization of bones. Rickets occurs in young animals in which the bones are actively growing. The equivalent condition in older animals is osteomalacia in which the osteoid matrix of the bones fails to calcify and the bones become progressively weak and liable to fracture. Phosphorus deficiency may induce similar lesions though many clinical outbreaks involve a complex mixture of causative factors.

Subclinically, vitamin D deficiency causes reduced productivity. In particular, the appetite decreases and there is poor weight gain and disappointing milk yield. Infertility is also said to occur.

Clinical signs and diagnosis

Non-specific signs include poor productivity, stunted growth and lameness. As the deficiency progresses clinical rickets supervenes with poor mineralization and low density of bones, which tend to bend and fracture easily. The joints enlarge and the growth plates thicken with uncalcified cartilage and osteoid.

Assay of vitamin D in the blood is seldom undertaken as a diagnostic procedure because the test is difficult to carry out. However, other secondary abnormalities in blood chemistry can give helpful guidance. For instance, plasma alkaline phosphatase is usually high in vitamin D deficiency as a consequence of the bone pathology. Calcium and phosphorus levels are low indicating defective absorption of minerals. Perhaps the most important question is differential diagnosis to rule out complicating factors such as protein, phosphorus and copper deficiency, or even fluorine toxicosis. A comprehensive metabolic profile test may be recommended in all cases of doubt.

Prevention and treatment

The control of vitamin D deficiency depends on the circumstances. The easiest choice is to allow adequate exposure to sunlight or to ensure that enough preformed vitamin D is fed. Vitamin D_3 is rarely given parenterally to control a deficiency, though of course it is commonly injected in massive doses to prevent milk fever (see Chapter 2, p. 24).

A special problem may be experienced with calves reared indoors. Milk itself usually contains sufficient vitamin D. Calves fed replacer diets may need supplementary oral doses of 20–45 IU/kg body weight daily. Animals with clinical signs usually take time to recover after treatment, depending on the extent of the lesions, though rapid restoration of appetite is usually achieved.

Excess vitamin D is toxic. It involves excessive drinking (polydipsia) and copious excretion of urine (polyuria). Continuously heavy dosing with vitamin D induces metastatic calcification of blood vessels, the heart wall and the kidney tubules.

Vitamin K

Introduction

Cattle rarely suffer from vitamin K deficiency because ample supplies occur in most plants, and microbial activity in the rumen synthesizes still more. An exception occurs in 'sweet clover disease', a condition caused by a secondary deficiency of the vitamin due to vitamin K antagonists found in certain plants and silage.

Vitamin K is so-called because Danish scientists first called it 'koagulation factor'. Deficiency of it results in faulty coagulation of the blood and in potentially fatal haemorrhages.

The cause

During spoilage of hay and silage, coumarins, which are relatively harmless compounds normally found in certain plants such as sweet clover, are converted to the toxic dicoumarol, a potent vitamin K antagonist. This induces vitamin K deficiency which prevents the synthesis of prothrombin and possibly other coagulating factors in the blood. Dicoumarol can cross the placenta so that newborn animals may suffer from haemorrhages as well as the mother cow.

Vitamin K deficiency has been reported in individual cattle suffering from obstruction of the bile duct—the absence of bile inhibits absorption of the vitamin. Also, a vitamin K deficiency has been suggested to explain why certain calves bleed heavily after simple surgery such as castration or dehorning, but the evidence remains meagre. Finally, another possible cause of vitamin K deficiency follows from the accidental consumption of rat poison which contains dicoumarol.

Clinical signs and diagnosis

All the clinical signs of vitamin K deficiency or 'sweet clover disease' stem from faulty blood coagulation and the resulting haemorrhages. Much depends on the quantity of dicoumarol consumed—some animals consume variable amounts over long periods but show no obvious ill effects. Others show stiffness of the limbs due to bleeding in muscles or joints. Still others develop large swellings or haematomas together with bleeding from the nose or the anus. Death follows if the loss of blood is massive.

Diagnosis can be confirmed by the detection of a prolonged blood clotting time or even by direct measurement of a low prothrombin content of the plasma.

Prevention and treatment

The obvious method of prevention is to avoid access to the toxic dicoumarol. This means that spoiled silage made from sweet clover should not be fed. However, some new strains of clover have now been bred which are free from coumarin.

Treatment involves correction of the prothrombinaemia with a transfusion of blood taken from a healthy animal which has not consumed the spoiled silage. Synthetic vitamin K (menadione) can then be given intramuscularly to restart the production of pro-thrombin.

Vitamin E

Although most natural feeds for cattle contain ample supplies of vitamin E it is rapidly oxidized and destroyed in old hay or silage and moist stored grain. Vitamin E performs a vital function in preventing the accumulation of toxic peroxides on cell membranes. In deficiency, nutritional muscular dystrophy results. In this re-spect the vitamin acts in concert with the trace element selenium, which is a molecular component of the enzyme glutathione per-oxidase.

The details of both vitamin E and selenium deficiencies are described in Chapter 8, p. 100.

Vitamin B

Introduction

Deficiencies of the vitamins of the B complex do not normally occur in cattle because the ruminal bacteria synthesize all of them, the only constraint being that the synthesis of some requires another factor, e.g. cobalt for vitamin B_{12} (see Chapter 8, p. 98).

Special diets given to young calves before ruminal function starts sometimes induce deficiency, but as milk normally contains sufficient it is only certain milk replacers that normally need supplementation.

Another situation associated with deficiency of the vitamin B complex exists as a result of depression in activity of the ruminal bacteria, either with long-continued antibiotic treatment, or with certain types of malnutrition such as severe deficiency of protein. In these circumstances the problem may receive relief with vitamin B as contained in a yeast preparation given orally.

The cause

The cause of vitamin B deficiency may follow from a simple deficiency, from enzymic destruction of the vitamin in the rumen, or from the absence of a co-factor essential in the ruminal synthesis. The following summarizes the position for each of the B vitamins.

Thiamine deficiency. Simple deficiency rarely occurs. However, the disease known as cerebrocortical necrosis is induced by the action of a thiamine antagonist (thiaminase) present in certain plants such as bracken (see Chapter 11, p. 133 for details). Another thiamine antagonist occurs in ensiled raw fish, which is a rarely-used by-product of the fishing industry in some countries.

Riboflavin deficiency. This deficiency never occurs in adult ruminants which are well able to synthesize their own supplies with the aid of the ruminal bacteria. Pre-ruminant calves on experimental replacer diets can show signs of deficiency which include poor appetite, diarrhoea, excessive salivation and lachrymation. The deficiency is not seen under practical conditions.

Nicotinic acid deficiency. This condition has not been reported even experimentally in pre-ruminant calves.

Pyridoxine deficiency. Although not seen under practical conditions it can be reproduced experimentally in calves. Affected animals show poor appetite and restricted growth with anaemia. This progresses to nervous signs with convulsions.

Pantothenic acid deficiency. This does not occur normally in cattle, but it can be induced experimentally in calves which develop skin lesions (dermatitis), poor appetite and reduced growth. In advanced cases demyelinization of nerves ensues with nervous signs.

Biotin deficiency. This can be produced experimentally by long-continued oral dosing with antibiotics. The deficiency causes paralysis of the hindlegs and possibly skin lesions also.

Folic acid deficiency. This has not been observed under practical conditions. The deficiency in humans causes anaemia and thus this might be expected in cattle but no evidence for it has yet been uncovered.

Choline deficiency. This has been induced experimentally in calves. The affected animals become weak and gradually recumbent. It is said that choline, added to the diets of growing steers, improves their daily weight gain, but this, of course, does not necessarily imply a pre-existing deficiency.

Vitamin B_{12} or cyanocobalamin deficiency. This is caused by deficiency of the trace element cobalt which is an essential component of the vitamin's molecular structure. For details of this deficiency see the section on cobalt (Chapter 8, p. 98).

Clinical signs and diagnosis

Only two of the vitamin B deficiencies occur under practical situations, namely cerebrocortical necrosis or thiamine deficiency, and vitamin B_{12} deficiency due to low intake of the trace element cobalt. These are described in Chapter 7, p. 87 and Chapter 8, p. 98. All the others might occur on unusual diets, especially in young calves which have not yet developed ruminal function. Clinicians should be on the alert for unusual clinical signs linking with exotic feeds. These signs might not be highly specific but amount merely to unexpected inappetance. Alternatively, a veterinary surgeon might be asked to advise on the use of a new feed. The possibility of a vitamin B complex deficiency should always be borne in mind.

The emergence of a new problem commonly stimulates a new method for diagnosis, often based on a test for an enzyme or a metabolite which is affected by the vitamin. Examples include the transketolase test developed for thiamine deficiency and the methylmalonic acid and FIGLU tests for vitamin B_{12} deficiency.

Prevention and treatment

Precise diagnosis of vitamin B deficiencies can usually be followed by rational and effective supplementation.

Vitamin C

Vitamin C, or ascorbic acid, is not normally deficient in cattle, or even in young calves. It is synthesized in the tissues and is not thought to be a dietary essential. However, recently a skin disease of young calves correlated with a low concentration of plasma ascorbic acid was reported, and furthermore it responded to parenteral ascorbic acid. Is this evidence of a possible deficiency? The situation needs further investigation.

10 / Congenital disorders

Introduction

The so-called metabolic disorders of cattle usually result from the stress of high production coupled with unusual or inadequate diets. These are more properly called 'production diseases'. This contrasts with the situation in human medicine where metabolic diseases are true errors of metabolism, or congenital abnormalities of individuals who lack a key enzyme, or suffer from a block in an important metabolic pathway. Disorders of this kind occur in cattle also. A surprising number of breeding cattle carry undesirable and defective genes, possibly in a hidden form, so that they fail to be recognized. Most of these abnormal genes are recessive in character and are not expressed in the heterozygote. This means that the problem only comes to light when two carriers are mated and the resulting homozygous calves express the trait in a clinical form.

The breeding of animals has a disadvantage in that it relies on selection from comparatively few, high-quality animals. Only a limited number of bulls stand at stud producing the semen used in artificial insemination and should one of them be a heterozygous carrier then the defective gene could become spread widely before it was realized. The situation worsens if the bull's semen is stored and used to inseminate his daughters who may then give birth to homozygous offspring which show the clinical effects of the genetic defect.

Fortunately the danger is appreciated. All breeding animals at stud receive close scrutiny for undesirable genetic traits. Families of affected bulls can be traced back and eliminated from future breeding stock. Even so, congenital abnormalities present a serious risk. The disease of mannosidosis is a good example. It lay dormant in Angus cattle for several years until some herds in New Zealand contained as many as 35% carrier cows, originating it is believed from one carrier bull. A new test had to be developed to detect the affected stock and prevent further dissemination of the trait.

Congenital defects can arise spontaneously by genetic mutation. They lie dormant, perhaps indefinitely, until a critical point is reached in intensive breeding so that they become expressed as clinical disease.

Not all congenital defects inflict disease. Some confer benefit. For instance, glucose-6-phosphate dehydrogenase deficiency of red blood cells in Hereford cattle protects against trypanosomiasis and other blood-borne protozoal parasites.

The main need is for specific diagnostic tests. Then eradication becomes straightforward. Furthermore, continued watchfulness is essential to identify any new congenital diseases before they have time to spread in the population.

An important point needs emphasis. Many genetic traits are complex and not expressed in terms of a single error of internal metabolism, but as interacting factors in nutrition or in endocrinological make-up. Many of these traits are suspected but few can yet be identified with precision. It is known, for instance, that milk fever susceptibility is in part inherited but no single defective gene or metabolic abnormality has yet been detected which is responsible for the effect.

Each of the major metabolic disorders will be described in turn.

Mannosidosis

Introduction

This is a lethal disease of certain Angus and Murray Grey cattle. It is associated with deficiency of an enzyme, α-mannosidase.

The cause

The defect expresses itself as a storage disease involving an error in glycoprotein metabolism. The stored material is an oligosaccharide containing mannose which would normally be metabolized by the enzyme α-mannosidase. The oligosaccharide cannot be metabolized in affected calves and thus it accumulates in vacuoles, especially in the brain cells which eventually degenerate, provoking nervous signs.

Clinical signs and diagnosis

Affected calves become progressively incoordinated. They show a characteristic 'head nodding' sign, become unthrifty and die within a year.

Diagnosis depends on a blood test for α-mannosidase. Carriers usually have half the normal concentration of the enzyme, whereas clinically affected stock have only very low levels.

Prevention and treatment

Prevention involves the eradication of animals with the genetic defect. There is no treatment.

Glycogenosis

Introduction

This disease resembles mannosidosis being due to deficiency of an enzyme, α-glucosidase, in beef shorthorn cattle.

The cause

The defect is an inherited recessive trait which involves failure to metabolize glycogen, which then accumulates in various cells of the body especially those in the muscles, heart, liver and brain. Affected cells undergo degeneration with progressive loss of function.

Clinical signs and diagnosis

Affected calves show poor growth, progressive muscular weakness, incoordination and eventual recumbency.

Diagnosis depends on detecting the lack of α-1, 4-glucosidase activity in lymphocytes.

Prevention and treatment

If control measures are put in hand an eradication scheme based on the diagnostic test would be the only valid option. There is no treatment.

GM1-gangliosidosis

Introduction

This defect is another inherited storage disease known to occur in
Friesian cattle. It involves a genetically-induced lack of an enzyme
β-galactosidase.

The cause

The lack of enzyme causes the progressive accumulation of ganglioside in tissues which undergo cellular degeneration and loss of
function, especially in the brain.

Clinical signs and diagnosis

Progressive loss of mobility occurs as the nerve cells become
infiltrated with ganglioside. Blindness supervenes owing to lesions
in the retina and optic nerve.

Diagnosis involves ophthalmoscopic examination to detect the
abnormal retina. Also lack of β-galactosidase can be detected in
several cells including blood leucocytes.

Prevention and treatment

If needed, the enzyme test could be used to identify affected stock
so that an eradication policy could be implemented. There is no
treatment.

Inherited achondroplastic dwarfism

Introduction

This is a genetic defect associated with massive anatomical abnormalities of the head and limbs. Abnormalities of the thyroid occur
and there seem to be defects in other body functions.

The cause

The defect appears to have originated from breeders' attempts to
produce blockier, shorter-legged beef animals. Thus, unconscious-

parakeratosis develops progressively. There is poor growth rate. The thymus is hyperplastic.

The defect responds to oral supplementation with zinc. There is an impairment in zinc absorption (see Chapter 8, p. 104).

11/Disorders associated with toxic factors

Fluorosis

Introduction

New bone has the capacity for the temporary sequestration of toxic elements such as fluorine. Unfortunately, long-continued excess intake of fluorine leads to toxicity resulting in severe and painful bone disease (see Chapter 2, p. 33). In addition to osteoporosis and osteomalacia, the teeth become mottled and there is excessive wear of developing teeth.

The cause

Fluorosis is a chronic disease usually caused by the ingestion of small amounts of fluorine in the diet or in drinking water. Fluorine is present naturally in rock, often in association with phosphate, and thus soils and surrounding water can contain large amounts of fluorine, even as high as 8.7 ppm in water. Although most surface water contains little fluorine, that from deep wells or artesian bores can contain much larger quantities. However, levels of fluorine likely to be toxic to animals are not usually encountered in natural circumstances. Plants absorb little fluorine and thus little is ingested from pastures.

Top dressing of pasture with phosphatic limestone is a common cause of fluorosis and larger quantities may be ingested if animal feeds are supplemented with cheap rock phosphate, particularly if this is done to counteract phosphorus deficiency.

Pollution by fumes and ash from industrial plants does occur, although legislation to control this is now general.

However, even small quantities of fluorine ingested over a long period can exert effects due to the ability of bone to adsorb fluorine thus leading to bone disease.

Clinical signs and diagnosis

Fluorine is a general tissue poison. If large amounts are ingested then death rapidly ensues following gastric irritation due to the formation of hydrofluoric acid. Nervous signs and tetany may follow the drop in calcium levels in the serum when inactive calcium fluoride is formed. Blood clotting may also be inhibited.

In cases of chronic intoxication there is a decrease in appetite, probably due to reduction of activity in the rumen. However, the mottled appearance of the teeth may be the first clinical sign. Exostoses may develop where the fluorine is deposited on the periosteal surface. Calcium and phosphorus are excreted rapidly in the urine and then rapidly mobilized from skeletal reserves to restore normal blood levels, with resulting osteomalacia and osteoporosis (see Chapter 2, p. 33).

Normal cattle have blood levels of up to 0.2 mg/dl of fluorine and 2–6 ppm of fluorine in urine. Higher levels may not reflect intake but occur as a result of deposits already in the body. Serum calcium and phosphorus levels are usually normal, but there is a significant correlation between the amount of fluorine fed and alkaline phosphatase levels in the serum.

Bone lesions can be detected by radiographic examination. There may be increased porosity or thickening of compact bone and narrowing of the marrow cavity. Biopsy samples of ribs can be used for accurate determination of fluorine content.

Prevention and treatment

The content of water supplies should be tested. If levels are high the addition of slaked lime will reduce the fluorine content. Dressing of pasture with phosphatic limestone and the addition of rock phosphate to feed should be avoided.

There is no treatment, although calcium salts can be given intravenously to replace the precipitated calcium in the serum. Adequate supplies of calcium and phosphorus will also help to facilitate storage of fluorine in the bone for the present.

Calcinosis

This is caused by the consumption of *Trisetum flavescens*, or yellow oat grass, which contains toxins having vitamin D activity.

The condition is characterized by extensive metastatic calcification and is described in Chapter 2, p. 37.

Drunken calf syndrome—alcohol poisoning

Introduction

Drunken calf syndrome can follow excess energy intake. The predisposing condition is the presence of glucose and absence of animal fat in the diet. This can occur in newborn calves given a diet of fat-free milk to which glucose has been added. The production of alcohol from these conditions causes a drunken staggering gait and may be followed rapidly by other signs of intoxication, and can sometimes culminate in death.

The cause

The production of alcohol is due to fermentation of the glucose in the rumen by a naturally occurring yeast *Torulopsis glabrata*. This multiplies rapidly in the rumen of young animals and ferments any glucose to produce large quantities of ethanol, up to 500 mg/100 ml of stomach contents. Newborn animals have little ability to metabolize ethanol as they have low levels of alcohol dehydrogenase in the liver. Also, young animals are especially susceptible to intoxication when the alcohol is absorbed into the blood.

The fermenting yeast does not metabolize sucrose or lactose, and thus the disorder is confined to animals receiving replacer diets containing hydrolysed starch.

Clinical signs and diagnosis

The staggering gait and incoordination are characteristic signs of the condition.

Prevention and treatment

Prevention relies on giving a better milk replacer diet in which hydrolysed starch is not the only source of energy.

Copper poisoning—excess copper intake

Introduction

Acute copper poisoning usually occurs as a result of accidental administration of copper salts. Chronic copper poisoning can occur in areas where the soil is naturally rich in copper, although the amount of copper present in the pasture plants will depend not only on the copper content of the soil but also the amount of molybdenum and sulphate, which affect the absorption of copper. In areas of molybdenum-rich shales there is little likelihood of excess copper intakes. However, some plants do aid the retention of even small amounts of copper, whilst others such as *Heliotropum europaeum* cause excessive copper retention following liver damage.

The cause

Excess copper salts may be ingested when feed is contaminated. Plants may be contaminated with fungicidal sprays, and water may contain copper from parasiticide drenches or when snail eradication programmes are in progress. Pasture may also contain excess copper after dressing with copper salts to correct a copper deficiency. In industrial areas pollution with copper is possible. Feeding seed grain which has been treated with antifungal agents, as well as mineral mixtures containing excess copper may also contribute to excess copper intake.

Parenteral injections to correct copper deficiency should be checked to ensure that excessive doses are avoided.

Clinical signs and diagnosis

As soluble copper salts are protein coagulants, the ingestion of excess amounts causes intense irritation of the alimentary mucosa. Thus severe gastroenteritis accompanied by abdominal pain and severe diarrhoea are the immediate clinical signs. Severe shock follows accompanied by a fall in body temperature and increased heart rate. Collapse and death may follow within 24 hours. In calves that survive the illness, haemoglobinuria and massive haemorrhages occur.

Small amounts of copper ingested over a longer period of time show little effect, but the copper accumulates in the liver. This may take up to 6 months to reach maximum levels, but when the copper is released into the blood the animals become acutely ill and die very quickly.

In these cases there is usually no disturbance of the alimentary tract function, but thirst, haemoglobinuria and jaundice appear suddenly. Death is ascribed to acute anaemia and haemoglobinuria nephrosis. Methaemoglobinaemia is often present and packed cell volume drops from 40% to 10% in 48 hours.

Liver biopsies are the only way to determine whether there is liver damage, and copper levels may be determined from the material.

A mean copper level of 0.07 mg/l is suggested as normal. Two methods of ascertaining copper amounts are available: either estimation of caeruloplasmin, which correlates well with blood copper, or the erythrocyte superoxide dismutase test which may be preferred (see Chapter 8, p. 97).

Prevention and treatment

Care should be taken to avoid excessive administration of copper, whether by incorrect dose rates or when applying copper dressings to pasture to correct a copper deficiency. Feeding seed grains treated with antifungal agents, and plants contaminated with copper-containing fungicidal sprays should be avoided. Water containing parasiticide drenches may contain toxic amounts of copper.

In particular, it is important to avoid access to such plants as *Heliotropum europaeum*, *Senecio* spp. and *Echium plantagineum* which specifically affect the retention of copper, or cause increased affinity for copper in the damaged liver cells.

The application of molybdenized superphosphate to pasture (70 g of molybdenum per hectare) increases the molybdenum content of the pasture and reduces the retention of copper.

It is also suggested that the avoidance of stress and malnutrition is important in preventing outbreaks.

In acute cases gastrointestinal sedatives and symptomatic treatment for shock are recommended. In chronic cases, the provision of additional molybdenum in the diet is recommended for sheep, though this has not been used in cattle.

Dicoumarol poisoning

Sweet clover poisoning is caused by the ingestion of hay containing sweet clover (*Melilotus alba*). This contains coumarol as a natural constituent, which can be converted to dicoumarol through the action of moulds. The toxic effects of dicoumarol, which is a vitamin K antagonist, are described in Chapter 9, p. 114 (vitamin K deficiency).

Nitrate and nitrite poisoning

Introduction

The problem of ammonia poisoning due to sudden excess consumption of urea has been described in Chapter 7, p. 89. A similar toxic effect occurs when animals are turned out onto fresh grass with a high content of soluble protein which can ferment so rapidly that ammonia poisoning ensues.

A related problem of nitrate poisoning occurs when grazing animals are turned out onto pasture which has been fertilized with high levels of nitrates, especially if this has been done during dry weather, when plant growth is restricted and the levels of nitrate remain high. Alongside is the problem of nitrite poisoning; nitrite is formed from nitrate in the plant either before or after ingestion.

The cause

Cereal crops can contain toxic amounts of nitrate, particularly after repeated dressings of nitrogenous compounds and especially if crude sewage is applied. Although ensiled material contains less nitrate than the fresh crop, the juices produced during ensilage may contain toxic quantities of nitrate and should be avoided. Hay made from nitrate-rich material usually retains that quantity of nitrate. In damp conditions the presence of moulds on the hay may convert the nitrate to nitrite.

Specific plants contain larger amounts of nitrate than others. Immature green oats, wheat, barley and hay may contain toxic amounts. Other plants such as variegated thistles (*Silybum marianum*) and winged thistle (*Carduus tenuiflorus*), *Astragalus* and *Oxytropis* spp. and mintweed (*Salvia reflexa*) can cause nitrite poisoning and resultant heavy losses in cattle. Linseed grass (*Urochloa panicoides*) is also poisonous, containing 5.5% nitrate in its stems. Some plants can accumulate nitrate, particularly if rapid growth follows a drought period when nitrate dressings have remained on the pasture.

Water from deep wells may contain nitrate levels of 1700–3000 ppm, especially if filled by seepage from highly fertilized soils.

Clinical signs and diagnosis

The predominant sign of nitrite poisoning is dyspnoea with rapid respiration due to anoxia. The anoxia is caused by the formation of methaemoglobin when the nitrite is absorbed. Nitrites also act as vasodilators and so can contribute to the tissue anoxia. As with ammonia poisoning some clinical signs originate from derangement of the central nervous system. There is excessive salivation, muscle tremors and incoordination, followed by tetany and death.

In cases of nitrate poisoning the clinical signs may be delayed for 6 hours, the time required for conversion of nitrate to nitrite. Early signs include abdominal pain, diarrhoea and vomiting, and excessive salivation. Death occurs in cattle when blood levels of methaemoglobin reach 9 g/100 ml blood.

In cases of nitrate poisoning post-mortem examination reveals evidence of gastroenteritis. In nitrite poisoning the blood is dark red or coffee coloured. Petechial haemorrhages are present in the heart muscle and there is much vascular congestion.

Blood samples collected during life can be used to estimate nitrite by the diphenylamine test. Methaemoglobin can also be detected by using reverse spectrometry, but only if the sample is collected less than 2 hours before testing. In the field, a modified diphenylamine reagent provides a qualitative test which can also be applied to test probable toxic plant material. However, these tests can give inaccurate results.

Specimens for laboratory examination should include blood for methaemoglobin estimation, ingesta and plant material. Cerebrospinal fluid can be removed for analysis at post-mortem but must be collected within 2 hours of death.

Prevention and treatment

Ruminants should be fed an adequate carbohydrate diet and care should be taken to avoid pastures that contain dangerous plants, or which have been heavily fertilized recently, especially if the weather has been dry and plant growth restricted by lack of water. When cattle are at pasture the feed should not contain more than 1% nitrate.

Silage or hay which may contain high levels of nitrate should be restricted, in particular hay which has been stored in damp conditions.

It is also important to avoid supplying water known to contain high levels of nitrate.

Methylene blue injected intravenously at a dose rate of 20 mg/kg is recommended for treatment of cattle. If much toxic material has been ingested then the dose may need to be repeated in 6–8 hours. In small doses the methylene blue rapidly converts methaemoglobin to haemoglobin, though in large amounts it can itself cause methaemoglobinaemia.

Bracken poisoning and thiamine deficiency

Introduction

Bracken fern poisoning is highly fatal in cattle, but as the intake of bracken has to be large, the number of deaths are usually small. Cattle do not eat bracken readily but young fronds may be appetizing if forage is scarce. Some samples of hay can contain toxic amounts and if bracken is used as bedding this may be eaten.

The cause

Although the toxic factor in bracken poisoning has not been identified, its effect is to cause thiamine deficiency. For details of thiamine deficiency and the associated disease, cerebrocortical necrosis or polioencephalomalacia, see Chapter 7, p. 87. Thiamine deficiency can be detected by the erythrocyte transketolase activity and treatment undertaken. However, administration of thiamine, vitamin B_{12} and folic acid do not prevent the occurrence of the effects of bracken poisoning.

Clinical signs and diagnosis

In ruminants bracken poisoning is usually associated with depression of bone marrow activity and pancytopenia. There is increased capillary fragility, prolonged bleeding time and defective clot retraction. In calves this clotting defect appears to be due to the formation of heparinoid substances and the presence of toxic amines in the blood.

Clinical signs of this type of bracken poisoning occur in 2–6 weeks after eating the bracken. There is high fever, dysentery or melaena, and bleeding from the nose, eyes and vagina. There is increased heart and respiratory rate and death ensues in 1–2 days.

Blood examination showing decreased numbers of erythrocytes and leucocytes will confirm the diagnosis.

Prevention and treatment

To avoid bracken poisoning cattle should not be allowed access to bracken in large quantities.

Where the numbers of erythrocytes and leucocytes are much reduced in numbers blood transfusions are recommended.

Selenium poisoning

Introduction

Selenium poisoning occurs in areas where the selenium content of the soil is high, where certain specific plants which retain selenium are present in pasture, or where accidental overdoses are given. The affected animals may become blind and show nervous signs such as head pressing, though in chronic cases of poisoning there is emaciation, lameness and often loss of hair.

The cause

Selenium-rich soils are mainly found in North America and Australia, and the incidence is greatest where specific selenium-selecting plants are present in the pasture. These plants, *Astragalus* spp. and *Oxytropis* spp. in North America and *Morinda reticulata, Neptunia amplexicaulis* and *Acacia cana* in Australia are good indicators of the high selenium content of the soil.

The effect of selenium ingestion is influenced by the cobalt and protein status of the animal. If either of these are deficient then susceptibility to selenium increases. Cattle are less susceptible than sheep, but selenium in feeds should not exceed 5 ppm dry matter, and feeding on pastures containing 25 ppm dry matter for several weeks can cause chronic poisoning. Acute poisoning can follow grazing on pasture containing 2000–3000 ppm of selenium.

Selenium is given to treat cases of enzootic muscular dystrophy and, as stated in Chapter 8, p. 103, it is important to check the dose rate, as 1 mg/kg body weight can kill and lesser doses can cause acute poisoning. Excessive amounts may also be given if selenium is added to the diet to correct selenium deficiency.

Clinical signs and diagnosis

In acute poisoning there is respiratory distress, watery diarrhoea, fever and tachycardia. Often there is abnormal gait and posture leading to prostration, and death may then soon follow.

Two forms of chronic poisoning occur. One is known as 'blind staggers'. This usually displays nervous system involvement with a staggering gait, blindness and then paralysis and finally death due to respiratory failure. The other form is expressed as ill-thrift. Here there is dullness, emaciation, a rough coat and hair loss, and lack of vitality. Hoof abnormalities are also present and lameness is often severe. As selenium can cross the placental barrier newborn animals may show hoof deformities.

In acute cases post-mortem examination reveals congestion and necrosis of the liver as well as congestion of the renal medulla. The rumen is impacted and may show areas of ulceration. In accidental poisoning there is extensive damage to the liver, lungs and myocardium.

In chronic selenium poisoning there is atrophy and dilation of the heart, necrosis of the liver and glomerulonephritis. There is also erosion of the articular surfaces.

Selenium can be detected in the urine, hair and milk. Clinical illness occurs when selenium levels are above 4 ppm in urine and over 5 ppm in hair. Blood levels should not exceed 3 ppm. Estimation of selenium-containing enzymes, e.g. the glutathione peroxidase of erythrocytes, gives a measure of selenium in the blood. Selenium can also be measured in abattoir specimens.

Prevention and treatment

Access to selenium-containing plants should be avoided. In particular, care should be taken where selenium has been added to the diet to correct a selenium deficiency. Doses of selenium for injection should be carefully checked.

A high-protein diet has a general protective effect, and oral administration of copper is said to be an effective preventive measure. There is no specific treatment.

12 / Interactions

Introduction

Many metabolic and nutritional disorders fail to fit into the main definition. A diverse group of miscellaneous conditions exist which remain non-specific in their clinical effects. These have a very definite basis in nutritional or metabolic abnormality, or in interactions between several abnormalities. Because of their key positions in the metabolic pathways the alimentary tract, the liver and the skeleton are involved in these conditions. These include infertility, bone disorders and indigestion.

Infertility

Doubtless most problems of infertility simply relate to lack of proper timing between insemination and ovulation. This is a matter for husbandry and bears no relationship to nutritional or metabolic disorders. Nevertheless, so many nutritional defects involve infertility as a clinical sign that the subject deserves special treatment. Basically it is a multifactorial problem.

Many investigators link infertility with poor energy intake or, more precisely, to factors such as declining body weight or hypoglycaemia. There is little doubt that diets low in energy lead to negative nutritional balance in early lactation coupled with low blood glucose. Indeed, various strategies for the measurement of blood glucose have been proposed as monitoring systems to indicate fertility. Many consider that the actual concentration of blood glucose at service is of less importance than the changes which have taken place beforehand; a falling concentration being undesirable but a rising value indicating optimal fertility. This observation requires further thought. In an earlier chapter it was stated that blood glucose may not reflect energy status directly but a decline in liver function and gluconeogenesis (see Chapter 6, p. 73). For instance, fatty change in the liver shows a clear correlation with infertility. The severity of liver pathology links with hypoalbuminaemia, cholesterol, bilirubin and certain liver-specific enzymes. In other words, low blood glucose is merely one of many signs that all stem from failing function of the liver. In fact, liver failure with impairment of fertility can be detected even before calving. This fits in with the discovery that even mild subclinical ketosis with elevated β-hydroxybutyric acid in the blood correlates with relative failure to conceive.

Trace element deficiencies correlate with infertility. Blood copper levels link with fertility. Copper deficiency is a multifactorial problem causing anaemia, low yields of milk and increased number of services to conception and delay in conceiving after parturition. Supplements of copper reverse the situation. Selenium too affects fertility in a similar way. In addition, manganese deficiency impairs fertility—again restored by dietary supplementation. Surveys of cobalt (vitamin B_{12}) deficiency have shown clear links with infertility, though in this case the effect might have been mediated by poor appetite and subclinical ketosis. Finally, it must not be forgotten that multiple trace element deficiencies frequently interact. Surveys of farms for infertility frequently reveal a high incidence of multiple deficiencies requiring supplementation with more than one element.

Mineral intake relates to infertility. Many investigators have noted deficiency of phosphorus and hypokalaemia with infertility. However, the situation is very complex. Sodium states too are important, possibly linked with inappetance and indigestion. However, some excess intakes may impair fertility, e.g. excess phosphorus, potassium, calcium and also protein. The precise reason for this remains obscure. Clearly the situation is complex. An excess of one mineral or trace element leads to inhibition of absorption of another and vice versa. The objective must surely be the achievement of an appropriate balance.

Several factors stand out in relation to fertility. First, the liver holds a central position in metabolism and any factor interfering with liver function will probably have a secondary effect on conception and fertility. Second, in high-yielding cows much depends on a continuity of input. This will depend not only on an adequate and suitable diet, but also the ability of the alimentary tract to digest and absorb the nutrients required. Lack of appetite, gut stasis as well as toxic factors will disrupt this supply and lead to negative nutritional balance. In addition, reserve supplies from the skeleton may well be required to maintain the normal blood levels of minerals that cannot be supplied in sufficient quantities from the diet.

Thus a complex series of factors lead to infertility and any treatment must depend on the complete evaluation of the interacting systems.

Bone disorders

These are another group of conditions which result from metabolic disorders. The lack of minerals required for normal bone development may derive from an inadequate or unsuitable diet, from inadequate absorption from the alimentary tract, or by being diverted to another more pressing metabolic need. This is illustrated by the diversion of calcium from skeletal needs to that of milk production. Excess availability of minerals can also cause problems, as for instance where excess calcium causes osteopetrosis. There is also competition between needs for, and excess of, the minerals calcium, phosphorus and magnesium. The factors controlling these conflicting demands, and the resultant bone disorders are described in Chapter 2, p. 32.

Indigestion

The importance of the alimentary tract, and particularly the rumen, in metabolic disorders is outlined in Chapter 1, p. 3. Any interference with the functioning of the tract has serious consequences as it disrupts the supply of vital nutrients and metabolites. Indigestion is an ill-defined condition, but is involved in and consequent upon many other disorders.

Acute indigestion itself may lead to diarrhoea and subsequent dehydration (see Chapter 4, p. 52). In addition, cattle secrete copious quantities of saliva and the contained water must be recirculated by resorption of the water further down the alimentary tract if the animal is not to become dehydrated. Therefore, any disruption in the flow of ingesta through the tract can lead to dehydration. Flow disruption can arise from a foreign body in the oesophagus, abomasal torsion or displacement, or be due to bloat.

When the indigestion is due to overeating the osmotic pressure of the ruminal and intestinal contents may suddenly increase.

Ruminal contents are normally at a lower osmotic pressure than the blood and thus water is absorbed passively through the rumen wall. This flow of water is rapidly reversed if large quantities of highly fermentable food in the rumen cause a rise in osmotic pressure. This reverse flow of water again results in dehydration. Haemo-concentration is said to be characteristic of acute indigestion.

In addition, if large amounts of highly fermentable carbohy-drates are fed to cattle the large quantities of lactic acid produced as a result of fermentation can lead to a rise in acid conditions within the rumen. This sudden rise in acidity can give rise to inappetance and indigestion as well as to systemic acidosis. The disorder of metabolic acidosis is described in Chapter 6, p. 75.

Indigestion is also associated with the feeding of large amounts of urea. This is often used as a cheap substitute for protein. Not only does it cause indigestion, but if too rapidly hydrolysed the amount of ammonia produced can lead to ammonia poisoning (see Chapter 7, p. 89).

In many cases of indigestion, impaction, tympany and rumini-tis due to the feeding of high concentrate rations, the more disastrous consequences can be avoided by allowing sufficient time for the animal to adapt to the new diet.

The causes of subclinical and chronic disorders of the ali-mentary tract may be more difficult to determine, but bacterial infection and the presence of parasites will affect the normal functioning of the alimentary tract.

Ageing and longevity

There is little known about the effect of age on the occurrence or severity of metabolic disorders. Such evidence as exists suggests that older animals exhibit a slowing down in metabolism. Globu-lins increase with age and this may reflect the gradual acquirement of immunity over a lifetime of exposure to antigens.

The occurrence of parturient paresis rises with age from 0.2% in initial calvings to over 9.6% at the 6th or subsequent calvings. There is a slowing down of bone metabolism and decreased absorption from the gut. The amount of exchangeable calcium in the skeleton also decreases with age as well as the rates of exchange of calcium ions between the blood and various storage com-partments of the body. Excretion of calcium in the faeces also increases. This is probably due to a slowing down in the rate of flow of intestinal contents. In older cows there is also a severe dip in blood haemoglobin and packed cell volume following parturition.

It may be expected that repeated experience of metabolic disorders such as milk fever, mild ketosis, and fatty liver will have effects in the longer term. However, little is known of the effects of metabolic disorders on ageing or longevity as animals are usually culled when productivity declines at a relatively early age.

13 / Conclusions

The metabolic disorders that arise from changes in the dynamic equilibrium of body systems have been described in this book. Such disorders occur as a result of inadequate or unsuitable input of body requirements, breakdown in homeostatic systems such as endocrine control, insufficient availability of enzymes, or when there is an excessive outflow of metabolites to meet the demands of production. The metabolic stability of the animal also depends on the efficient functioning of the alimentary tract, in particular the rumen, the capacity of the liver to produce many of the components needed for lactation, and the presence of sufficient mobilizable reserves of minerals in the skeleton or body tissues for use in times of short-term deficiency.

The disorders themselves may also interact to cause conditions such as infertility, indigestion and bone disorders, all of which are associated with decreased productivity.

It was suggested in Chapter 1, p. 3 that the term 'production disease' might be used to describe metabolic disorders, as many of the disorders in animals do result from a breakdown in the animals' capacity to meet the demands of high production.

Productivity is measured in terms of growth rate, milk and meat production as well as the production of young animals to replace the adult stock. Breeding of selected stock has produced high-yielding milk cows and double muscled beef stock, and systems for rapid growth of calves, earlier conception rates and the production of twins all contribute to increased productivity.

However, if these demands of increased productivity are to be met then the input of the necessary nutrients must be adequate. The lack of available calcium in the high-yielding milk cow at parturition results in milk fever. Likewise the input must be in a suitable form. Highly fermentable concentrate rations can increase the energy input for cattle but metabolic acidosis may result and, similarly, feeding cheap protein in the form of urea may cut feeding costs but it may also cause ammonia poisoning.

Good husbandry is also essential to prevent the occurrence of metabolic disorders. Most cattle obtain their supplies of minerals and trace elements from the pasture they graze. Some soils are deficient in some of these such as iodine, copper and sodium, and these deficiencies must be corrected. However, the effects of over-dressing of soil with copper, or excessive use of nitrogen fertilizers can themselves cause copper or nitrate poisoning. The lack of a suitable and adequate water supply will result in dehydration.

The metabolic disorders resulting from the increased demands of high productivity and the ways in which correct husbandry can prevent such disorders are described in this book.

There still remain problems associated with subclinical and chronic conditions that reduce productivity, as well as the effect of repeated episodes of metabolic disorders such as milk fever and ketosis on the future productivity of the animal and its lifespan. These need further investigation.

The diagnosis, treatment and prevention of metabolic disorders will increase productivity. However, in countries where droughts occur frequently and there are poor soil conditions the input of essential nutrients is often inadequate. The resultant metabolic disorders do not just reduce productivity, but there is actual loss of milk and meat for the local population, as well as the loss of replacement animals for future years. In these conditions the correct diagnosis, treatment and prevention of these problems prove their worth.

Efficient cost-effective productivity of milk and meat remains important in the agricultural economy and avoidance of metabolic disorders will reduce some of the costs. These costs will also include that of suffering to the animal itself. Not only should this be avoided for the animal's welfare, but an ill animal does not produce as well as a healthy one.

New systems of agriculture and production will no doubt make further demands on cattle and new metabolic disorders will be recognized. Further investigations are needed to increase our knowledge and ability to recognize and overcome the disorders as they arise.

Index

acetonaemia *see* ketosis
achondroplastic dwarfism 122–3
acidosis 62, 140, 142
adrenal corticosteroids 46
adrenocorticotrophin hormone
 (ACTH) 69, 72
ageing 140–1
 and calcium absorption 12
 and fatty liver syndrome 141
 and ketosis 141
alanine 82, 86
albumin 83, 84
alcohol poisoning 128
alimentary tract 3–4
 obstruction of, and electrolyte
  metabolism disorders 62–3
alkaline phosphatase 106, 113
amino acids 82–3
ammonia poisoning 4, 89–90, 140, 142
anaemia
 and copper deficiency 96
 and iron deficiency 93–4
antidiuretic hormone (ADH) 46, 62
ascorbic acid deficiency 118

baldy calves 124
'biological ceiling' 6
biotin deficiency 117
'blind staggers' 135
blindness 109, 110
boglame *see* osteoporosis
bone disorders 32–40, 139
bone metabolism
 and calcium homeostasis 13
 and magnesium homeostasis 15
bracken poisoning 133–4
Brassica and iodine deficiency 91
butyric acid 64, 66, 71

caeruloplasmin 37, 97, 130
calcinosis 127
calcitonin 1, 39–40
 and hypocalcaemia 19
calcium
 concentration in blood 9
 control by calcitonin 1, 10, 11, 39–40

endocrinological control of 1, 11–12
factors affecting absorption of 12
input/output relationship 11–12
and lactation 4, 5, 13
pool size of 2
calcium borogluconate 17, 18, 21, 24–5,
 74, 79
calculi formation
 in urolithiasis 41–3
carotene 108, 109, 110
 as vitamin D antagonist 112
C-cells 11, 19, 39–40
cerebrocortical necrosis 87–8, 116, 117,
 133
Cestrum diurnum 38
chief cells 10
chloride and alimentary tract
 obstruction 62–3
cholecalciferol *see* vitamin D_3
choline deficiency 117
citrate as magnesium chelating agent 29
cloprostenol 24
cobalt 95
 and rumen function 85
cobalt deficiency 71, 73, 96
 and infertility 138
 and vitamin B_{12} 98–100, 116
congenital disorders 119–25
copper
 absorption of 5
 and liver necrosis 6
copper deficiency 5, 37, 94–8
 and anaemia 96
 cause 95–6
 clinical signs and diagnosis 96–7
 and infertility 38
 prevention and treatment 97–8
copper poisoning 97, 129–31, 143
corticosteroids, adrenal 46
creatine 102
creatine phosphokinase (CPK) 26, 102
'creepers' 26
cruban *see* osteoporosis

dehydration 45, 49–54
 due to diarrhoea 52–4, 139